Jefferson Barela
Erica P. Neves
Gabriel H.C. Bonfim

Standardizing burn care

Jefferson Barela
Erica P. Neves
Gabriel H.C. Bonfim

Standardizing burn care

In industries and power plants by occupational nurses

ScienciaScripts

Cover image: www.ingimage.com

This book is a translation from the original published under ISBN 978-3-330-77176-5.

Publisher:
Sciencia Scripts
is a trademark of
Dodo Books Indian Ocean Ltd. and OmniScriptum S.R.L publishing group

120 High Road, East Finchley, London, N2 9ED, United Kingdom
Str. Armeneasca 28/1, office 1, Chisinau MD-2012, Republic of Moldova, Europe
Managing Directors: Ieva Konstantinova, Victoria Ursu
info@omniscriptum.com

Printed at: see last page
ISBN: 978-620-8-63845-0

SUMMARY

1 INTRODUCTION

When we talk about occupational nursing care in industrial or plant outpatient clinics, we immediately recognize the care given to polytraumatized patients. In many cases, these types of incidents involve large injuries spread across the body, which can affect all three layers of the skin, as well as muscles and bones in more serious cases. Therefore, the approach to initial care for such injuries needs to be systematized in order to facilitate and standardize the procedures to be carried out.

In general, especially in cases of injuries that involve disfigurement and incapacity of the individual, both in pre-hospital care services and in emergency rooms, standardization is essential to ensure that future complications do not occur. It is clear that it is of substantial importance for professionals to analyze and recognize all the possible injuries that the individual may have, and not to focus exclusively on treating burns, which are more obvious.

It is important to know that a burn of any size can be a serious injury, and the timely application of simple emergency measures minimizes the morbidity and mortality of these injuries.

Therefore, the aim of this study is to verify the quality of nursing care provided by specialist nurses in outpatient units of industries and plants to employees injured by burns. To this end, a bibliographical survey was carried out in which it was possible to highlight an update and a perspective, with the compilation of studies by: Atallah, Cega, Schiavon, Kikuchi and Cavallazzi, 2004; Flavio Novaes, 2003; Gomes, Serra, Guimarâes, 2001; Hudak and Gallo, 1997; National Safety Council, 2002; Smeltzer and Bare, 2002; Soares, Almeida, Gonçalves, 1996; Taborda, 2004; Tocantins, Gomes, 1988; Soares, 1998; Knobel, 2006 and Santos, 2007.

2 LITERATURE REVIEW

2.1 Burns

2.1.1 Physiology and Pathophysiology

Burns are traumatic wounds caused, in most cases, by thermal, chemical, electrical or radioactive agents, which act on the lining tissues of the human body, causing partial or total destruction of the skin and its attachments. Depending on their severity, they can reach deeper layers such as subcutaneous cellular tissue, muscles, tendons and even bones (GOMES et al. 2001, p.151).

Integral skin is one of the most important elements in protecting the human body from environmental aggressors. The balance of the microbiota is altered after a burn, allowing pathogenic bacteria to establish themselves and grow. The proliferation of these bacteria in a favorable environment (susceptible host) can culminate in sepsis, a complication that accounts for around 75% of deaths in patients with severe burns (TOCANTINS, 1988, p.40-56).

The clinical manifestation of a thermal lesion will vary from a small blister (flictena) to more serious forms, capable of triggering systemic responses proportional to the extent and depth of these lesions (GOMES and SERRA, 1999, p.333).

The main aim of treating thermal injury is to restore the damaged tissues, either by second intention healing or by autografting. Unfortunately, these two processes don't occur very quickly and various disorders require equal attention and commitment if therapeutic success is to be achieved (GOMES and SERRA, 1999, p.333).

2.1.1.1 Pathophysiological Sequence

For a correct therapeutic approach to burn patients, knowledge of the pathophysiological process of thermal trauma is of fundamental importance, in order to understand the speed of the whole process and its different stages (SOARES et al.p1996).

It can be seen that a burn is a dynamic trauma that can affect all organs, with the extent and duration of organic dysfunctions proportional to the extent of the injury. In minor burns, there is only a local relationship, while in moderate and severe burns, there is an exuberant local reaction, accompanied by severe systemic repercussions. The changes are biphasic, with an early hypofunction of the systems, followed by a later hyperfunction (GOMES and SERRA, 1999,p.333).

2.1.1.1.1 *Hemodynamic response*

With thermal trauma, collagen is exposed in the affected tissue and, consequently, histamine is activated and released by mast cells. This causes an increase in capillary permeability (APC), which in turn allows the passage of plasma filtrate into the interstitium of the affected tissues, which can cause both tissue edema and significant hypovolemia.

When activated, the kallikrein system (blood protein systems) produces kinins which further contribute to APC, aggravating tissue edema and hypovolemia (GOMES and SERRA, 1999, p.333).The kinins and the exposure of collagen activate the phospholipase-arachidonic acid system, releasing prostaglandins, especially prostacyclin (PGI2), further increasing capillary permeability.

Another activated pathway is thromboxane, which, together with circulating plasmin and thrombin, causes a deposit on the walls of these capillaries, causing an increase in hydrostatic pressure of up to 250%, further contributing to tissue edema (GOMES et al., 1995. p.192). Making an analogy: it's as if the body's firefighters were turning on their hoses, drenching the tissues in an attempt to put out a fire, causing a tremendous flooding of the affected compartments.

It should be noted that normal capillaries generally do not allow the passage of a single albumin molecule with a molecular weight of 60,000, however, after thermal trauma, molecules with a nuclear weight of up to 250,000 are able to pass through the capillaries (NOVAES, 2003, p.56-61). This phenomenon is temporary, lasting on average between 18 and 24 hours, with the maximum peak of increased permeability around 8 hours after the injury, and then regressing to its normal state.

In normal tissue, capillary pores allow crystalloid solutions to pass through in both directions, contributing to a perfect balance with the tissue interstitium. These pores do not allow colloid solutions, whose molecular weight exceeds the diameter of the capillary pores, to pass through (GOMES and SERRA, 1999, p.333).

The increase in capillary permeability allows not only crystalloid solutions but also colloid solutions to pass through. This process can cause significant edema in the affected tissues, as well as an increase in the colloidosmotic pressure of these tissues, mainly due to the colloids, consequently causing water retention.

This phenomenon has a strong impact on the burn patient's therapeutic resuscitation, since it is recognized that crystalloid solutions should be used and colloids avoided for as long as the PCA lasts, thus minimizing the occurrence of edema (MARINI and WHEELER, 1999, p.1403-1419). Despite this, a significant amount of colloid is retained in the capillary pore after it returns to its normal diameter, causing tissue edema.

Using cellular micropipetting techniques, an increase of 2,000 to 4,000% in interstitial suction force has been described, which will further increase and facilitate the tissue flooding described above. Only a few years ago it was proven that the APC of burned tissues only occurs in burned tissue and that the edema observed in non-burned tissue is also due to an acute reduction in the plasma colloidosmotic pressure of the burned patient (Soares et al., 1996).

After the burn, there is contraction of the intravascular compartment and depletion of energy reserves, culminating in metabolic acidosis, which rapidly evolves into hypovolemic shock. All this pathophysiological knowledge has had a direct impact on the therapeutic approach to burn patients, reformulating not only the quality but also the quantity of fluids used in the resuscitation of these patients from shock. Another point that differs from the therapy carried out in the years

40,50 and 60 is that formulas are no longer used to replace the burn victim's shock, and only the quantities needed to maintain a satisfactory urine output and stable hemodynamics are infused (TOCANTINS, 1988, p.40-56).

2.1.1.1.2 *Immune System Response*

After a burn, the patient usually presents with secondary immunodeficiency, which can be aggravated by many factors, such as: age; geographical location; nutritional conditions; and, of course, the extent and depth of the injuries;

Firstly, thermal injury causes a loss of integrity of the skin or mucosa, which acts as a mechanical barrier to microorganisms. There is also a physiological response with local vasodilation, APC and leukocyte chemotaxis at the site of the injury. There is an activation of factor XII of the coagulation system which alters the expression of adhesion molecules (ICAM-1, CD11 and selectins), causing microvascular thrombosis with the release of vasoactive substances such as serotonin, leukotrienes and prostaglandins. The phagocytic capacity and bactericidal activity of neutrophils also decrease, which has been linked to an increase in the frequency of infections. It seems that these infections may be associated with bacterial multiplication within neutrophils, where the bacteria would be protected from antibiotics (GOMES, 2001, p.151).

As a result of the injury, altered substances from the skin enter the circulation, creating an influx of antigens that will be presented by macrophages, inducing the formation of suppressor cells. Arachidonic acid metabolites are released, such as prostaglandins and leukotrienes. Prostaglandin E-2 induces the proliferation of suppressor T cells and also increases the suppressor activity of macrophages. PGE-2 stimulates bacterial endotoxins, which enter the bloodstream from external and internal sources of Gram-negative bacteria, causing excessive production of thromboxane, generating ischemia and thrombosis (TOCANTINS, 1988, p.40-56).

The complement system is also activated, and C3A and C5A concentrations are reduced, influencing the host's defense due to their ability to produce an inflammatory process with cell chemotaxis, opsonization and positive stimuli to phagocytic cells capable of destroying the invading agent. There is also the release of active biological products which cause tissue and cell damage. It is postulated that a decrease in plasma levels of C3 leads to consumption opsoninopathy, removing the stimulus for the migration of defense elements to critical areas of inflammation (GOMES et al, 2001, p.151).

At the same time, there is a large decrease in serum fibronectin, which seems to be associated with an increase in the frequency of infections due to reduced opsonization.

In humoral immunity, there is a decrease in the concentration of immunoglobulins, which seems to predispose to sepsis. Gomes et al; 1995 suggest that the capacity of B lymphocytes to synthesize immunoglobulins remains normal, but the production of specific antibodies decreases after injury. IgG and IgA are the most altered and, 48 hours after thermal injury, plasma IgG levels of less than 500mg are predictive of sepsis. Interleukin 6, which promotes the terminal differentiation of B lymphocyte cells and the growth and differentiation of steam cells and hemolytic cells, can also show increased plasma levels (GOMES et al; 1995. p.192).

In cellular immunity, the main changes are associated with a decrease in the proliferative response, with alterations in the proportions between T helper cells and T suppressor cells. The increase in T cells reaches its peak around one to two weeks after thermal injury, and is directly related to the onset of sepsis. In practice, this change is determined by the count of Th and T cells, which is carried out using of the surface markers CD4 and CD8, respectively, where there is an inversion, i.e. CD8>CD4 (GOMES, 2001, p.151).

Currently, the main cause of immunosuppression in burn patients is a lack of interleukin2-producing cells. Associated with all these phenomena are cellular dysfunctions of the NK cells and antibody-dependent cellular cytotoxicity. All the immunological alterations are complicated by different clinical situations, such as: surgical procedures; anesthesia (thionembutal decreases the production of antibodies and nitric oxide); repeated blood transfusions (they stimulate the Ts lymphocyte); the use of antibiotics; the patient's nutritional state (GOMES et al; 1995. p.192).

2.1.1.1.3 Metabolic Response

The metabolic response to the injury is mediated by the hypothalamic-pituitary axis, with the release of agents such as interleukins, prostaglandins, tumor necrosis factor and leukotrienes (vasoactive mediators). The initial stage of the injury is considered the Ebb Phase ("reflux or shock"), which is characterized by hypometabolism, a decrease in cardiac output, oxygen consumption and basal metabolic rate. This phase occurs immediately after the injury, with the release of catabolic hormones and vasoactive mediators (GOMES and SERRA, 1999, p.333).

In a few hours (48-72 hours), the reflux phase gives way to the "flow or hypermetabolic" phase, increasing the need for substrates that need to be obtained from the patient himself through a marked catabolism, "auto-cannibalism". If this process is inefficient, the substrates must be supplied through adequate nutritional support.

The hypothalamic-pituitary response is characterized by a eurohormonal discharge, the main hormones being: antidiuretic (ADH), growth hormone (GH); adrenocorticotropic hormone (ACTH); and possibly thyroid stimulating hormone (TSH). While the rise in TSH and ADH may be transient, the fundamental effect of thermal injury is represented by a marked and permanent rise in cortisol, GH, catecholamines and glucagon. During the initial stages, insulin secretion seems to be inhibited or decreased due to the predominance of the alpha-adrenergic effects of adrenaline over its beta-adrenergic effects (GOMES et al., 2001, p.151).

Caloric expenditure and protein catabolism are higher in burns than in any other physiological stress. With regard to energy expenditure, this can be up to twice the normal value predicted for expenditure at rest, because it acts in favor of wound healing, hyperdynamic circulation, respiratory drive and protein flow. It is clear that the primary stimulus for this hypermetabolism is still uncertain in the field of research, but there is evidence that catecholamines are a "key factor" in the process. In the presence of a marked predominance of catabolic hormones, energy substrates are mobilized at a rate two to three times higher than normal (GOMES et al; 1995. p.192).

The stock of glucose in the form of glycogen is quickly used up, since granulation tissue depends predominantly on anaerobic glucose as its main source of energy. Liver and muscle glycogen is used up within a few days of the injury, requiring a mechanism to synthesize new glucose (GOMES et al., 2001, p.151).

Undoubtedly, one of the fundamental metabolic changes is the increase in the supply of glycogen precursors, including amino acids through protein catabolism. This is quite pronounced in the first few weeks of evolution, with a negative nitrogen balance lasting on average until the third week in the case of major burns. There is no effective weight gain until most of the lesions have been covered (SMELTZER and BARE, 2002, p.1432-1468).

Adipose tissue is also mobilized through the lipolysis of triglycerides. The free fatty acids produced are useful in gluconeogenesis, despite the persistent hyperglycemia of hyperinsulinemia, which partly limits the use of this substrate in energy production. Carnitine plays an important role in this process by facilitating the transport of long-chain fatty acids into the liver's mitochondria. High triglyceride levels, normal ketone body values and increased carnitine loss may suggest that most of the fatty acids metabolized by the liver are re-esterified into triglycerides and are not used as an energy source (GOMES, 2001, p.151).

Thus, the objectives of nutritional support for patients with thermal injuries contribute to minimizing protein losses during the initial stages of the injury, as well as increasing the synthesis of lean tissue during the convalescent period. Its provision should be considered one of the priorities in the treatment of burn patients (TOCANTINS, 1988, p.40-56).

2.1.1.2 Lung function after burns

Burns to the face and neck can lead to edema and airway obstruction, even when there is no inhalation injury. Thermal injury can cause mucosal edema, which worsens in cases of hyperhydration. In extensive injuries, regardless of the region affected, there may be changes in the airways similar to facial and neck burns, and airway edema may predispose to the appearance of atelectasis. At the same time, inflammatory mediators are released which can lead to the formation of non-cardiogenic pulmonary edema, intrapulmonary shunt and hypoxemia. Inflammatory lesions of the lung usually begin to appear from the third day of evolution, with a peak between the 7th and 10th day, which can lead to secondary severe respiratory failure and acute respiratory distress syndrome. This inflammatory phase is marked by hypermetabolism, which is associated with increased CO2 production and, consequently, increased respiratory work, which can precipitate the development of respiratory failure or worsen existing conditions (SMELTZER and BARE, 2002,p.1432-1468)

.

In deep, circular thermal injuries to the rib cage, edema, crusting and local retraction occur, most often causing restricted chest expansion and breathing difficulties. The occurrence of risk factors such as immobility, endothelial damage and changes in blood viscosity predispose patients to the appearance of thromboembolic phenomena (BOUNDY.2004.p.1014).

Inhalation injury is defined as the aspiration of superheated gases, steam or combustion by-products. This injury can lead to a reduction in airway caliber due to edema, bronchospasm, intrapulmonary shunt due to occlusion of small airways by endobronchial edema, reduced compliance due to alveolar collapse with alterations in the ventilation/perfusion ratio, loss of mucociliary clearance leading to tracheobronchitis and pneumonia. Respiratory failure, in cases of inhalation injury, may be due to a combination of factors (GOMES and SERRA, 1999, p.333.

The inhalation of smoke is invariably accompanied by the inhalation of carbon monoxide (CO), which is likely to be aggravated as it contains cyanide after the combustion of plastic components, culminating in the risk of poisoning. CO competes with oxygen for bonds with hemoglobin, but has 200 times greater affinity than oxygen. In addition, the presence of carboxyhaemoglobin increases the affinity of the heme radical, which is not occupied by CO, for oxygen, which hinders the release of oxygen into the tissues. Both changes in hemoglobin lower the partial pressure of tissue oxygen and have serious consequences for organs such as the heart and brain. When the partial pressure of tissue oxygen is low, CO binds to intracellular hemoproteins such as cytochrome c-oxidase, inhibiting their functions (GOMES, 2001, p.151).

The inhalation of hydrogen cyanide or cyanide gas, released from the combustion of plastics, silk and nylon fabrics, leads to an inhibition of cytochrome oxidase and, in general, of enzymes containing trivalent iron, thus determining an inability to use oxygen, lactic acidosis and cell death. Respiratory complications occur in around a third of patients who suffer major burns and are related to the majority of deaths (GOMES et al; 1995. p.192).

Respiratory failure can also be secondary to smoke inhalation, regardless of external injuries. The presence of inhalation injuries is an important indicator of severity, being a marker of clinical problems and death. The incidence of this type of injury varies greatly, being present in around 20% of patients admitted to burn treatment centers (GOMES et al; 1995. p.192).

2.1.1.3 Renal function after burns

With new knowledge about the pathophysiology of burns, mortality from hypovolemic shock has fallen sharply, even in major burn victims. Currently, hypovolemic conditions are seen in patients who receive late treatment due to delays in getting to hospital or delays in transfer procedures to a specialized center.

Acute ischemic or hypoxic tubular necrosis is what follows serious damage to the body, such as sepsis, major burns, polytrauma and shock of any etiology. The renal tubule is more sensitive to hypoxia than the glomerulus, due to its greater energy expenditure and less vascularization, with the segment of the loop of Henle being the most susceptible (SMELTZER and BARE, 2002, p.1432-1468).

In the initial phase of the burn, the great loss of water to the interstitium triggers the release of a large number of hormones such as catecholamine, aldosterone, angiotensin and vasopressin, which can lead to the pathogenesis of acute renal failure. It should be noted that hypovolemia can worsen the thickness of a burn, transforming a viable partial thickness into a full thickness, which contributes to morbidity and mortality (NOVAES, 2003.p.56-61).

Victims of electrical burns, charring or burns associated with crushing can develop acute tubular necrosis due to the direct renal action of the myoglobin degradation products released by the injured muscle. In the initial phase, after this type of injury, rhabdomyolysis occurs, releasing a large amount of myoglobin, as well as phosphorus and potassium, which is filtered and reaches the tubules. If there is low tubular flow, the pigment concentrates and can damage the tubular cells. The pathogenesis of kidney dysfunction in this condition remains unknown. Several mechanisms have been proposed, such as the direct effect on tubular cells of myoglobin degradation products containing iron ions, tubular obstruction, altered renal blood flow due to arteriolar vasoconstriction caused by myoglobin depleting intra-renal nitric oxide. This ischemia is often aggravated by the trauma itself.

Hemoglobin, when released in large quantities, as in the transfusion reaction, can cause acute tubular necrosis in a similar way to myoglobin. In a severely burned patient with muscle destruction, hemolysis is also likely to occur, which will certainly aggravate the kidney damage. These patients require greater water replacement, often associated with osmotic diuretics, in order to promote high urine output (GOMES, 2001, p.151).

Currently, acute renal failure is more common in the late stages and is often related to sepsis, forming part of multiple organ failure (TOCANTINS, 1988, p.40-56).

A table showing the physiology can be found in Annex 1: Physiological changes after burning.

2.1.1.4 Cutting a Burned Fabric

If you make a cut in a particular burnt tissue, you can see three distinct zones. The zone closest to the thermal coagulation agent or coagulation necrosis, where there is intravascular coagulation. In the part of the tissue immediately adjacent to this, a zone of stasis is formed, where deposits can be seen on the vessel walls. In the region most distal to the thermal agent, a zone of hyperemia is formed, where an area of vasodilation is observed (SMELTZER and BARE, 2002, p.1432-1468).

2.1.2 Calculation of Burned Area and Indicators for Hospitalization

Calculating the body area affected by thermal trauma requires caution and attention. It is worth noting that there is a tendency to overestimate the area of the body that has been burned, and to include regions with first-degree burns. However, these lesions are not clinically important and therefore should not be included in the calculation of the damaged area (SOARES et al. 1996). To this end, it is essential that the professionals involved, especially nurses, have knowledge of the types of injuries caused by damaging agents (HUDAK and GALLO, 1997, p.890-912).

2.1.2.1 Factors that Directly Influence Prognosis

There are many factors that directly or indirectly influence the prognosis and determine the greater or lesser severity of a burn. When determining the therapeutic approach for a burn patient, it is necessary to know important information about the patient and their injury. Two factors directly influence the prognosis of the burn: the depth of the injury and the extent of the burned body surface. The deeper and more extensive the burn, the more serious the patient's survival prognosis (TOCANTINS, 1988, p.40-56).

2.1.2.2 Rule of Nine

The "rule of nine" is the fastest method for assessing the extent of burns. Because it is quick, practical and easy to remember, it is often used in emergency rooms. Although it is not a very precise method, it can be used in emergencies as an initial projection of the extent of the burned area.

The method consists of dividing the body into multiples of nine and therefore determining values: the head is worth nine; each upper limb is worth nine; the anterior thorax is worth 18%; the posterior thorax is worth another 18%; each lower limb is worth 18%; and the perineum is worth 1%.

It is clear that in the case of children, especially those under 4 years of age, the "rule of nine" should be applied with some modifications since children do not have different partial body surfaces to adults. For this purpose, 1% of the head should be subtracted for each year over one year of age and 0.5% of each leg should be added for each year over one year of age. A child's body surface is considered to be similar to that of an adult from puberty onwards

(GOMES et al; 1995. p.192).

In 3rd degree lesions, at least 48 hours should be waited before a final assessment is made, as third degree lesions can take a long time to define. The calculation of the burned body surface area will be of fundamental importance not only for the burn patient's prognosis, but also throughout treatment (NOVAES, 2003.p.56-61).

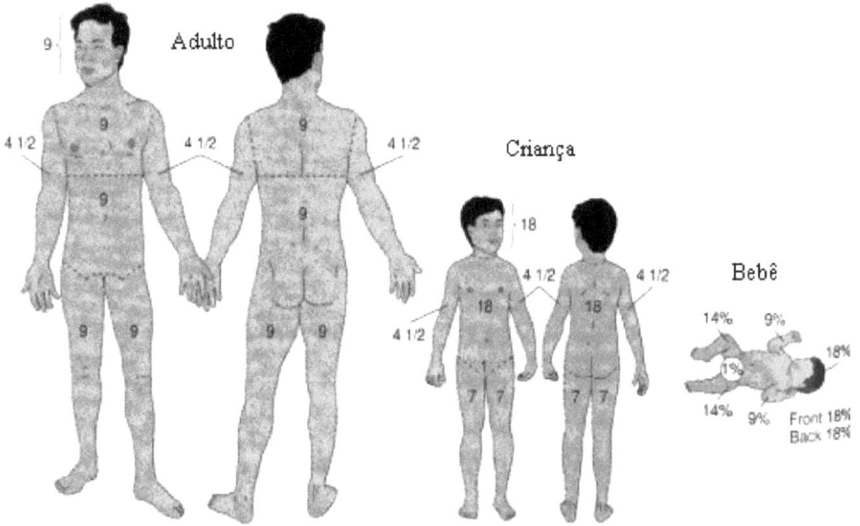

Source: http://www.ufrrj.br/institutos/it/de/acidentes/queima.htm

2.1.2.3 Lund - Browder scheme

The Lund-Browder scheme is one of the most accurate methods for defining the extent of burns, because it takes into account the proportions of the body in relation to age. In children, some regions, such as the head, may correspond to a much larger proportional area than in adults. When filling in the table, the value of each region affected should also be marked in relation to the degree of depth, so that an overall view can be taken of the percentage corresponding to 2nd degree injury, 3rd degree injury and the total percentage of body surface affected (NOVAES, 2003.p.56-61).

The extent of small, widespread burns can be calculated by comparing the size of the nurse's hand with the patient's hand. Taking into account the differences, the comparison will indicate that the palmar surface of an adult's hand is approximately equal to 1% of the adult's total body surface (HUDAK and GALLO, 1997, p.890-912).

Lund and Browder table:

Area %	*Age*				
	0-1	*1-4*	*5-9*	*10-14*	*ADULT*
Head	*19*	*17*	*13*	*11*	*7*
Neck	*2*				
Anterior/ Posterior Trunk	*13*				
Right/left arm	*4*				
Right/left forearm	*3*				
Right/Left Hand	*2,5*				
Nàdega Right/Left	*2,5*				
Genitalia	*1*				
Right/Left Thigh	*5,5*	*6,5*	*9*	*8,5*	*9,5*
Right/Left leg	*5*	*5,5*	*-*	*6*	*7*
Right/Left foot	*3,5*				

Source: http://www.saude.rj.gov.br/Queimaduras/classificacao.shtml

2.1.2.4 Degree of Burn

The depth of the burn depends on the causative agent, the time of exposure and the patient's previous conditions (SMELTZER and BARE, 2002, p.1432-1468). Its assessment involves determining the depth of the thermal injury to the skin, a process that challenges even the most experienced doctors. The greatest difficulty lies in classifying certain types of burns, such as electrical burns, which require a certain amount of time (2 or 3 days) for the injury to be truly defined. It is clear, however, that the most assertive assessment of depth can only be made by means of a histopathological study (biopsy).

In children, this will be even more difficult to determine, as their skin is much thinner than that of an adult, making them much more susceptible to deep injuries. For comparative purposes, it can be said that the same injury suffered by an adult can be much more severe and deep in a child (GOMES and SERRA, 1999, p.333).

In practice, differentiating between deep second-degree burns and third-degree burns is a major challenge for professionals. In addition, the presence of infection or severe hemodynamic instability can cause the injury to deepen, i.e. a superficial 2nd degree burn can evolve into a deep 2nd or 3rd degree. As a result, the first assessment should not be taken as the final one, and a reassessment should be carried out between 48 and 72 hours after the injury (SMELTZER and BARE, 2002, p.1432-1468).

Thermal injuries are classified according to three different degrees:

2.1.2.4.1 *1⁰ Degree Injury*

A 1st degree lesion is one that affects the outermost layer of the skin, the epidermis. Clinically, the lesion is hyperemic, moist, edematous and very painful. It does not cause hemodynamic changes, nor is it accompanied by significant clinical alterations, which is why the percentage of this type of burn is not included in water replacement calculations; it resolves in approximately five to seven days. Example: sunburn (GOMES, 2001, p.151).

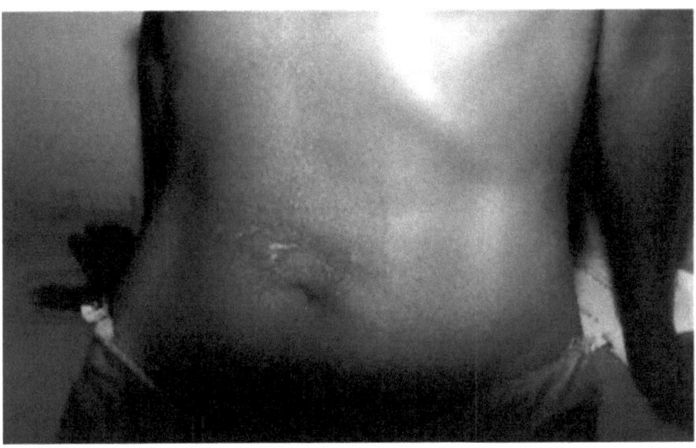

http://www.saude.rj.gov.br/Queimaduras/classificacao.shtml

2.1.2.4.2 *2nd Degree Injury*

It affects both the epidermis and part of the dermis. The most striking clinical feature is the formation of blisters or flictenas, which can be whole or ruptured. They can be differentiated into superficial and deep 2nd degree areas (SMELTZER and BARE, 2002, p.1432-1468).

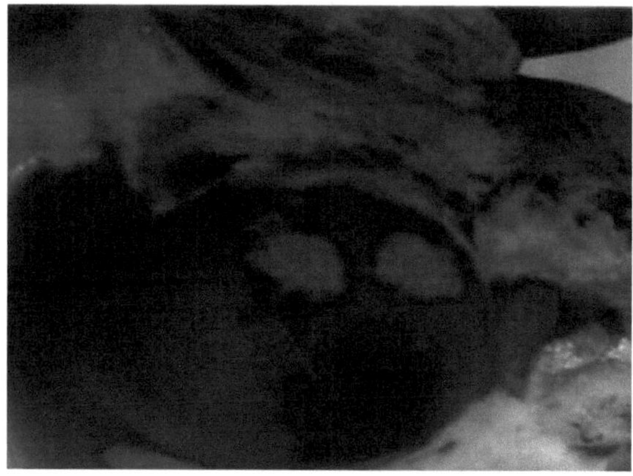

Source: http://www.saude.rj.gov.br/Queimaduras/classificacao.shtml

2.1.2.4.2.1 Superficial 2nd Degree Burn

They are also called partial thickness burns, affecting the entire epidermis (upper part of the skin) and part of the dermis (lower part of the skin), while retaining a reasonable amount of hair follicles and sweat glands. Clinically, they are characterized by the formation of flictenas, erythema, humidity and marked pain. When broken, the flictenae may show a pink, moist surface in superficial 2nd degree lesions, and a whitish surface with little shine in deep 2nd degree lesions (SMELTZER and BARE, 2002, p.1432-1468).

Superficial partial-thickness burns typically progress to total skin restoration in 14 to 21 days, with minimal scar formation. Example: Superheated liquid injury (GOMES et al; 1995. p.192).

2.1.2.4.2.2 Deep 2nd Degree Burn

Deep partial-thickness burns involve the destruction of almost the entire dermis and are closer to third-degree burns, with a paler color and less pain, as well as greater systemic repercussions. Although they may progress to restoration after three weeks, the newly formed epithelium is very friable, with recurrent ulceration and a strong tendency to hypertrophic scarring and the formation of contractures. The usual treatment for deep 2nd degree areas can involve tangential excision and skin grafting. Example: injury by superheated liquid, immersion or direct flame (GOMES, 2001, p.151).

2.1.2.4.3 *3rd Degree Injury*

It affects all layers of the skin (epidermis and dermis) and, in many cases, subcutaneous cell tissue, muscle and bone tissue. Clinically, it has a whitish or marbled appearance, accompanied by a reduction in tissue elasticity, which makes the tissue stiff. It may show thrombosed blood vessels. It is the most serious of all thermal injuries, causing deforming lesions. It can be electrical or thermal. Some authors consider charred areas to be "4th degree" injuries (GOMES, 2001, p.151).

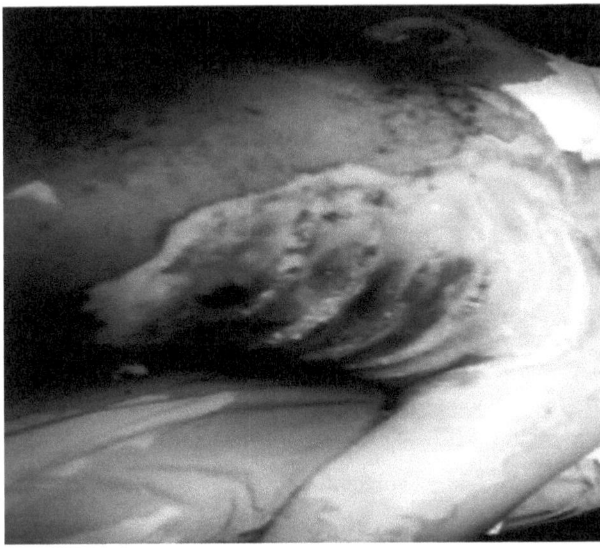

Source: http://www.saude.rj.gov.br/Queimad. shtml

In Annex 5: Burn depth table

2.1.2.5 Classification of burns

After assessing the depth and extent of the injury, we can classify burns according to severity into

2.1.2.5.1 *Mild burns*

1st degree - any length.

2nd degree - less than 10%.

3rd degree - less than 2%.

Most of the time they can be treated on an outpatient basis, do not lead to hemodynamic repercussions and rarely get worse (NOVAES, 2003.p.56-61).

2.1.2.5.2 *Moderate burns*

2nd degree - between 10% and 20%.

3rd degree - between 3% and 5%.

These patients require daily monitoring and can be treated on an outpatient basis, but most of the time it is more prudent to hospitalize them and observe the evolution of the clinical manifestations and the lesion (NOVAES, 2003.p.56-61).

2.1.2.5.3 Severe burns

2nd degree - exceeding 20% of the body surface area.

3rd degree - exceeding 10% of the CS.

In the case of critically ill, hemodynamically unstable patients, they need to be admitted to a burns treatment center or an intensive care unit (NOVAES, 2003.p.56-61).

2.1.2.6 Hospitalization Indications

Regardless of age, priority for admission to a burns intensive care unit should be given to major burns, with an area of more than 20% of the injured surface. Smaller areas of damage should be assessed by the Burn Unit team to check the need for hospitalization (SINDICATO DOS EMPREGADOS EM ESTABELECIMENTO DE SERVIÇOS DE SAÚDE DE BAURU. 1999).

As previously pointed out, the seriousness of a burn is determined mainly by the extent of the area of the body involved and, to a lesser degree, by the depth of the burn. However, other factors should be considered as aggravating factors, such as: the causal agent; pre-existing illnesses; trauma associated with other burns; the patient's age.

In the case of children under the age of two and a half and adults over the age of 65, the prognosis is usually more alarming, and therefore caution is recommended during their assessment and treatment, especially in order to avoid overvaluing symptoms and injuries. Clarification for family members and guardians is essential at this stage. In young children, this severity is not so noticeable, with a slightly better prognosis (TOCANTINS, 1988, p.40-56).

When the patient is transferred to the burns unit, a detailed medical report must be made of all the procedures and examinations carried out on the patient (NOVAES, 2003.p.56-61).

Hospitalization is indicated for the following types of burns:

A) 3rd degree lesion affecting more than 10% of the burnt surface.

B) Second-degree lesions affecting the upper area: 20% in adults and 10% in children.

C) Major burns to the face, hands and feet.

D) Perineal or genital burns (greater risk of contamination).

E) Circumferential burning of the extremities (due to constriction caused by edema, interfering with circulation).

F) Electrical burns (because they usually cause profound changes in acid-base balance and kidney failure) or chemical burns.

G) Airway burns.

H) Children under the age of two.

I) Concomitant systemic diseases (e.g. malnutrition).

J) Other associated traumas.

L) Impossibility of oral hydration (vomiting) (TABORDA et al.2004).

2.2 Pre-hospital and outpatient care in industrial units

Among the procedures intrinsic to pre-hospital care protocols, there are several stages, including checking the mechanism of injury (hit by a car, fall, electrical burn, fire, chemical burn, etc.) (NATIONAL SAFETY COUNCIL.2002.p.39-48). In addition, it is essential to assess the safety of the location (scene) where the victim was injured. The scene needs to be safe in order to provide care at the scene. If not, the first step will be to make the scene safe or remove the victim to a safe place. This measure aims to ensure the safety of the victim and the professional providing care (TABORDA et al. 2004). For example: when caring for victims of electrical burns, make sure that the source of electricity has been switched off. Care must be taken with victims of chemical burns, as contact with the product can cause burns to the professional providing the help (NATIONAL SAFETY COUNCIL.2002.p.39-48).

It is important to note that all professionals involved must use appropriate bio-protection devices (gloves, goggles) in order to be safe when approaching the victim and carrying out the primary examination. During this examination, the professional must assess the victim's level of consciousness using the AVDI method, which involves analyzing whether the victim is alert and able to respond to verbal and pain stimuli (AMERICAN HEART ASSOCIATION.2002).

The *Advanced Trauma Life Support Course* (ATLS) refers to the care of trauma patients, describing the stages of care. The first action involves checking the airways (A - airway). At this stage, care should be taken with regard to the occurrence of nasal vibrissae burns, the presence of carbonated sputum and a history of burns in a confined environment, which indicates smoke inhalation.

Signs of airway obstruction may not manifest immediately, which requires greater attention during the pre-attendance phase. Any patient with suspected carbon monoxide poisoning and/or inhalation should receive 100% humidified oxygen through a mask (ATALLAH et al.2004.p.668).

The progression of upper airway obstruction can be very rapid. Patients with pharyngeal burns, stridor or hoarseness have a high probability of developing upper airway obstruction and should therefore be intubated before being transferred. It is important that the tube is well secured, as there is a chance that it will no longer be possible to replace an endotracheal tube due to upper airway obstruction caused by edema (AMERICAN HEART ASSOCIATION.2002).

Once these precautions have been taken, guidance on the oxygenation of victims becomes paramount (B - Breathing). All patients with burns over 20% of their body surface area should be given 100% oxygen. At the same time, check the frequency and depth of breathing. Auscultate the chest. Tracheobronchitis with severe spasm and wheezing can occur both in the first few minutes and a few hours after the injury. Reassess the need for oxygen under mask, nebulization and intubation (AMERICAN HEART ASSOCIATION.2002). Third degree circumferential burns to the upper torso can impair ventilation and should be strictly monitored (GOMES, 2001, p.151).

After establishing airway patency, install venous access, preferably peripheral, with larger diameter catheters, or central access (**C** - Circulation). Start volume replacement with Ringer's lactate (2,000ml in boluses for adults and 20ml/kg for children). Install a bladder catheter to assess diuresis. Urine output should be kept between 30 and 50ml/h for adults and 1ml/kg/hour for children. The increase or decrease in the rate of hydration is defined by urine output (ATALLAH et al., 2004, p.668).

Most of the time, burn patients without inhalation injuries or associated head trauma are lucid and oriented, so it is advisable to observe the level of consciousness and assess whether there has been concomitant head trauma (**D-disability**). In cases of disorientation, this may be associated with hypoxia. Spinal injury should be assumed in all patients with a history of associated trauma and immobilization should be maintained until X-rays are obtained and fractures or dislocations are ruled out (GOMES, 2001, p.151).

The level of consciousness provides guidance as to the possible complications that may be manifesting themselves, such as: inadequate control of the infectious condition; hypoxemia due to pulmonary impairment or deviation of the hemoglobin saturation curve due to the presence of carbon monoxide; or changes resulting from head trauma that may be associated with the burn.

The presence of carbon monoxide poisoning implies a great variability of symptoms, so its serum dosage will be an additional parameter. Levels above 40% can determine alterations such as ataxia, cortical blindness and behavioral disorders, and levels above 50% can produce irreversible central nervous system damage (GOMES, 2001, p.151).

It is also advisable to remove the patient's clothing in order to slow down the burning process and to facilitate a complete assessment of the burned patient (**E** - exposition). Cooling the burned area is an important measure, but it only has value when applied immediately after the accident. If the patient is to be transferred, second-degree burns should be covered to relieve pain, and blisters should not be broken or antiseptic agents applied. Prophylactic antibiotics are not indicated immediately after a burn (MINISTÉRIO DA SAÙDE, 2002).

All rings, watches and other jewelry should also be removed from the affected limbs to prevent ischemia. Damage to the face, especially the eyes, should be checked (GOMES et al. 2001.p.151), and the head should be elevated to reduce edema in burns.

At the end of this examination, which lasts an average of two minutes, the professional carrying out the examination can conclude whether the victim is stable or unstable. If the victim is unstable, all the procedures should be carried out in the ambulance on the way to hospital, otherwise the professional can remain at the scene continuing the examination and carrying out the necessary procedures before removing the victim (HUDAK and GALLO, 1997, p.890-912).

The nurse's responsibilities include monitoring the inhalation injury and liquid resuscitation, as well as assessing the burn and vital signs, thus obtaining an accurate history and important guidance on the emergency measures to be taken (HUDAK and GALLO, 1997, p.890-912).

Blood pressure is not a reliable method of initial monitoring due to the exacerbated adrenergic response in the first few hours after the trauma, but it should be measured and recorded as an initial parameter. The detection of hypotension warns of the seriousness of the situation as well as co-morbidity.

It is clear that the heart rate is easy to access and guides the professional as to the appropriate water replacement at the time of circulatory rescue (GOMES and SERRA, 1999, p.333). In addition, cardiac monitoring is vitally important in order to detect cardiac rhythm and the presence of arrhythmias that could be lethal. It is therefore advisable, as far as possible, to carry out electrocardiographic recording, which can be done using defibrillator monitors.

Arrhythmias, such as ventricular afibrillation, asystole or ventricular tachycardia, are more frequent in accidents involving electric current and can be responsible for the sudden death of victims. It has been observed that certain electrocardiographic alterations, especially in young patients, give rise to suspicions of carbon monoxide poisoning (GOMES et al; 1995. p.192).

Generally speaking, the direct approach to the victim enables important data to be collected in order to define the procedures to be carried out. Therefore, as soon as possible, the history of the accident should be obtained from the victim themselves or their companion, verifying the causal agent, duration and seriousness of the injury. The anamnesis should then be directed towards obtaining the following information: context of the burn; causal agent; time of injury; environment of the event (closed or open); possibility of inaction; and associated trauma.

During this assessment, a second examination is carried out on the victim, called the "secondary examination". This, in turn, follows the same sequence as the primary examination, in order to reassess the victim, looking for problems that were not found and clarified during the primary examination (HUDAK and GALLO, 1997, p.890-912).

2.2.1 Secondary Exam

After the primary examination, burn care begins. In summary, the procedures include: cooling the burned areas with physiological solution or clean water and covering the burned areas with gas or dry compresses. It is clear that cooling the burned areas must be carried out immediately after the accident, otherwise it will lose its effectiveness. This, in turn, can be done by wrapping the victim in a sheet soaked in water, blocking the heat wave that acts on the burnt tissue for a certain period. There is no need to use cold water, since at room temperature it is already well below the temperature of the burnt tissue (TABORDA et al., 2004). It is important to protect the victim with a thermal blanket to avoid hypothermia.

When analgesics are needed, preference should be given to narcotics (morphine, meperidine), administered intravenously, paying attention to the risk of respiratory depression (PEREIRA, 2005). If there is any suspicion of damage to the airways or neurological impairment, the drug should be avoided (MINISTÉRIO DA SAÙDE, 2002).

During the initial care of a major burn patient, it is also important to identify symptoms and/or signs of trauma resulting from other factors, such as those occurring during an attempt to escape from a risky location. Falls from great heights can happen, especially during electrical burn accidents in a high-voltage area or network. In such circumstances, bone fractures and head and spinal injuries are not uncommon, as are pneumothorax, hemothorax, cardiac tamponade, chest fractures and other injuries (ATALLAH et al., 2004, p.668).

It's worth noting that a severe burn can contribute to seizures and is capable of causing more anxiety than pain itself.

2.2.2 Special Problems

2.2.2.1 Inhalation

Inhalation injury can consist of various physiological, pathological and clinical manifestations. It can occur in the upper airways, the tracheobronchial tree and/or the lung parenchyma. It is important to note that although the term inhalation injury is most often used broadly for all types of airway injury in burn patients, some authors use it to refer exclusively to lower airway injury (GOMES, 2001, p.151).

Inhalation injuries can be classified as direct thermal injuries and injuries caused by chemical agents. Direct thermal injury is caused by heat and steam and is usually limited to the supraglottic region (upper airways). Injury caused by chemical agents affects the lower airways and is most often caused by inhaling combustion products (smoke with its gases, aerosols and particles resulting from combustion or pyrolysis) (GOMES and SERRA, 1999, p.333).

With regard to treatment procedures, professionals are advised to evaluate the following aspects:

- Occurrence of singed nasal hairs;
- Burns of the oral and pharyngeal mucosa;
- Burns to the perioral area or neck;
- Expectoration of soot through coughing or a change in voice;
- History of being burned in a confined area (HUDAK and GALLO, 1997, p.890-912).

Some clinical studies carried out on animals have demonstrated the high efficiency of mechanisms designed to protect the lower airways. These include: rapid cooling of the air in contact with the upper portion of the respiratory mucosa and reflex closure of the glottis. These two mechanisms are usually sufficient to prevent thermal damage to the lower airways.

In general, heated dry air causes direct thermal injury to the upper airways and, less frequently, to the proximal portion of the trachea. It rarely causes injury to the lower airways. However, dry air heated under pressure, usually as a result of a strong explosion, can injure the lower airways, and in these cases the protection mechanisms are unable to prevent it. On the other hand, the simple inhalation of steam (moist heat), with a thermal capacity 4,000 times greater than heated air, can cause damage even to the lung parenchyma (HUDAK and GALLO, 1997, p.890-912).

In order to damage the respiratory tract, temperatures must be higher than 150°C. The temperatures found in smoke are usually between 260 and 280°C and only in special situations do they exceed 1,000°C (ATALLAH et al., 2004, p.668).

It should be noted that the heat from hot smoke, although not hot enough to cause direct thermal damage, is potentiated in the heated form (TOCANTINS, 1988, p.40-56).

Therefore, direct thermal injury is confined, in almost all cases, to the upper airways, and lower airway injuries, in turn, are produced by chemical agents through the inhalation of combustion products, with the exception of the following situations:

> Steam inhalation (moist heat/saturated heated air);

> Severe explosions (heated air under pressure that overcomes the reflex mechanism protecting the glottis);

> Accidents with fire and loss of consciousness with decreased glottic protection reflexes (GOMES, 2001, p.151).

Injuries caused by chemical agents can be divided into injuries caused by irritating asphyxiating agents (NOVAES, 2003.p.56-61).

Toxicological studies of fire victims recognize more than 50 inhaled chemical components and it is believed that only half of them have been identified (MARINI and WHEELER.1999.p.1403-1419).

Among the asphyxiating agents, CO (carbon monoxide) and HCN (hydrogen cyanide) poisoning are the most frequent causes of immediate death related to fires. CO results from the incomplete combustion of hydrocarbons or the combustion of cellulose (wood, paper, cotton) and is the main gas in almost all fires. It is an odorless, colorless gas with an affinity for hemoglobin 250 times greater than for oxygen, producing a drastic reduction in hemoglobin's ability to carry oxygen. HCN is found in insecticides, polyurethane foams and natural industrial products such as silk and wool. Its action is due to the inhibition of the cytochrome oxidase enzyme, which is essential for the utilization of O2 in cellular respiration (GOMES, 2001, p.151).

Irritants are largely responsible for so-called inhalation injuries. They vary according to the conditions of temperature, oxygenation and, in particular, the composition of the fuel. Chemical damage to the respiratory tree or lung parenchyma occurs when combustion products (toxic gases and/or carbonaceous material particles) are inhaled. These injuries are more frequent as a result of explosions of liquid or gaseous combustibles indoors or in fires where the victims are still present. There are a variety of combustion products that cause chemical damage to the lung parenchyma (GOMES eh SERRA, 1999,p.333).

The mechanism of inhalation damage due to the action of irritants is due to the production of diffuse epithelial damage in the respiratory tree, which can even compromise the epithelium of the lung parenchyma. The smoke is composed of toxic gases and suspended carbonaceous particles (ash). There is no evidence that the carbonaceous particles are harmful, but they are often coated with irritating aldehydes, ketones and organic acids that cause destruction of the tracheobronchial mucosa and a marked inflammatory response in the lung parenchyma (direct cytotoxic effect). They stimulate pulmonary macrophages which produce chemotoxic substances, with consequent leukocyte sequestration, release of proteolytic enzymes and free radicals. There is an increase in capillary permeability with extravasation of liquid into the alveolus and loss of surfactant, leading to pulmonary edema and focal atelectasis (SMELTZER and BARE, 2002, p.1432-1468).

The severity of the injury is largely determined by the degree of chemical solubility of the gases in water and lipids, as well as the duration of exposure (NOVAES, 2003.p. 56-61).

2.2.2.2 Clinical Manifestations of Inhalation Injuries

Acute asphyxia - when the victim is most often found at the scene of the accident as a result of inhaling asphyxiating agents, most frequently carbon monoxide (BOUNDY, 2004.p.1014).

Progressive obstruction of the upper airways - although thermal action in the upper airways alone can cause edema and obstruction, the inhalation of acrosols, acids and water-soluble irritants also leads to the formation of edema and inflammation of the oropharynx and larynx, manifested initially with hoarseness and later with respiratory stridor until complete obstruction (NATIONAL SAFETY COUNCIL, 2002.p.39-48).

Adult respiratory distress syndrome (ARDS) - chemical damage by irritants to the small airways and lung parenchyma manifests itself early (two to seven days) in the form of ARDS, or late (after the first week) as bronchopneumonia. The inhalation of combustion products into the intrathoracic airways develops an inflammatory process with damage and desquamation of the mucosa, inactivation of ciliary movements, formation of exudates and release of mucus and fibrin plugs, obstructing the smaller airways, with the formation of areas of atelectasis. The patient presents with a cough, retrosternal discomfort, chest tightness and wheezing. In addition, mucosal damage favors bacterial invasion and consequent bronchopneumonia. In the lung parenchyma there is an increase in circulating fluids and alveolocapillary permeability and the formation of pulmonary edema, which can evolve into ARDS. These factors are added to the pulmonary capillary damage that occurs even in isolation in the presence of skin burns in patients with large burn surfaces, through local activation of complement, neutropenia, local generation of free radicals and pulmonary capillary damage (ATALLAH et al., 2004,p.668).

Patients who inhaled heated air under high pressure or became unconscious and lost the reflex mechanisms protecting the lower airways may, although more rarely, suffer direct thermal injury to the lower airways and lung parenchyma, with the development of the pathophysiological mechanisms and clinical manifestations described above (SMELTZER and BARE, 2002, p.1432-1468).

Similarly, although not yet fully understood, it seems that there are long-term effects of inhalation injury. Chronic residual effects include bronchiolitis obliterans, tracheal stenosis and bronchiectasis (TOCANTINS, 1988, p.40-56).

2.2.2.3 Transportation

Sometimes transportation is a critical factor in resuscitating the victim. This decision should be made taking into account the resource capacity of the rescue team, including considerations such as time-distance and the intensity of the burns the victim has (TABORDA et al.2004).

In more advanced centers, there are professionals who specialize in transporting high-risk patients. If it is not possible to take the patient to a center of this type, it is recommended that it be carried out by health professionals with experience in intensive care who are qualified to carry out procedures and cardiopulmonary resuscitation, which can be a doctor and a nurse with these qualifications (ATALLAH et al., 2004, p.668).

Gomes (2001, p.151) reports that the factors involved in transporting a large burn are:

. Severity of injury and resources.

. Victim's condition.

. Transportation modes.

. Time-distance.

. Destination alternatives.

- Local treatment
- Emergency room
- Regional hospital
- General Hospital
- Burn Treatment Center (LTQ)

. Vehicles (GOMES et al. 2001.p.151).

2.2.2.3.1 Ambulance

It is recommended for short distances, a maximum of 200 km, avoiding greater risks for the patient and physical strain for the transport team. The patient must already have some kind of dressing and be hemodynamically stable. They are the most widely used vehicles, due to their cost and availability. Their disadvantages are the difficulty of accessing some places and the concentration of traffic in some regions (TOCANTINS, 1988, p.40-56).

2.2.2.3.2 Helicopter

It has the advantage of speed and ease of access, avoiding traffic congestion in large cities. Due to the vibrations, high noise levels and lack of space in the cabin, it should be used for very stable patients who are not at risk of requiring intubation or other more complex maneuvers. Their disadvantages are their high cost and limited radius of action, close to 300 km (GOMES, 2001, p.151).

2.2.2.3.3 Aviation

Their advantages are speed, lower operating costs than helicopters and a large radius of action. The disadvantages are the need to use airports and the combination of these transports with those carried out by land vehicles until they reach the CTQ. Airplanes without a pressurized cabin present turbulence, difficulty in maintaining cabin temperature, greater use of oxygen and the possibility of worsening certain pathologies, such as pneumothorax, due to the greater expansion of gases. Contensive dressing is mandatory. The changes in atmospheric pressure and the partial pressure of oxygen must be taken into account (GOMES et al; 1995. p.192).

Whichever vehicle is used for transportation, it is important to ensure harmony and easy access when distributing the equipment, as well as the height of the cabin in which the patient is transported, to make it easier to carry out procedures (SOARES et al. 1996).

Attention: It is much more prudent to hemodynamically stabilize a major burn patient, make sure there are no airway injuries, provide some kind of topical dressing, than to carry out an uncertain removal, without prior communication, without the patient being stabilized and without receiving any topical care. This rush to remove can have very bad consequences (GOMES and SERRA, 1999, p.333).

2.3 Basic Care in Emergency Care

2.3.1 Airways

As already mentioned, observing the respiratory pattern, maintaining a clear airway and ventilating the patient will always be the first steps taken by the first-aid doctor. It is not necessary for these patients, even when they have scorched nasal vibrissae, to be promptly intubated or tracheostomized, procedures which greatly increase the risk of complications such as pneumonia, pulmonary barotrauma, tracheal stenosis, among others. Clinical signs that suggest airway burns have a high incidence of false positives; for example, facial burns are present in 70% of patients with inhalation burns, but 70% of patients with facial burns have no airway damage. Hypoxemia may be absent in 80% of patients in the initial phase of care. Changes in auscultation, such as snoring, wheezing and rales, are rare (GOMES, 2001, p.151).

In patients with extensive burns and victims of accidents in closed environments, the first-aider must be alert to the possibility of airway burns, and the full arsenal for confirming the diagnosis must be used. In these patients, severe airway edema may develop, and if there is any doubt about the need for orotracheal intubation, it should be performed. Intubation should always be performed on patients with altered level of consciousness, assessed on the Glasgow scale as eight or below, to protect the airways from bronchoaspiration. If possible, bronchoscopy should be performed early for diagnosis and to help with difficult intubations (ATALLAH et al., 2004, p.668).

Patients with suspected or confirmed carbon monoxide poisoning should be given 100% oxygen, so that they can release carboxyhemoglobin from the red blood cells more quickly. The time needed for levels to fall by half is 4 hours if the patient is breathing ambient air, and less than 1 hour if they are receiving 100% oxygen (GOMES and SERRA, 1999, p.333).

Patients who have inhaled smoke need a greater amount of liquids in the first 24 and 48 hours, compared to those who have not (TOCANTINS, 1988, p.40-56).

2.3.2 Burn Shock

The next step is to observe the hemodynamic state. In the first moments after the burn, due to the large release of catecholamines, the patient often has normal or high blood pressure and is tachycardic. Therefore, heart rate and blood pressure are not ideal parameters for assessing the patient's volume status. Urine output should be monitored, as it is the most reliable parameter of tissue perfusion, and a delayed bladder catheter should be passed in a closed system (GOMES, 2001, p.151).

A peripheral vein in the non-burned area should be punctured with the catheter with the largest possible lumen diameter, in order to start volume replacement. If there is no puncturable vein on the entire surface, a catheter should be placed in the vein through the burned skin, since the wound is still sterile at this stage. Catheterization of the subclavian vein is often difficult due to hypovolemia and collapse of the vein, carries a high risk of pneumothorax and should be avoided. Upper limb vein dissection may be necessary when peripheral venipuncture is impossible and should not be delayed in any way (TOCANTINS, 1988, p.40-56).

Volume resuscitation should be instituted as soon as possible, preferably before the patient arrives at the hospital, when they are attended by emergency services. Otherwise, as soon as they arrive at the hospital, they should be given saline or hypertonic solution in the appropriate volume to achieve satisfactory urine output. Delayed resuscitation leads to high mortality, not only because of the development of hypovolemic shock, renal failure and metabolic acidosis, which would be the terminal complications of a patient who has been without hydration for hours, but mainly because of altered gastrointestinal perfusion. Studies have shown that thermal injuries induce ischemia, mediated by angiotensin II, and reperfusion injury in the intestine, leading to increased permeability and bacterial translocation. The translocation and absorption of bacterial endotoxins will be responsible for sepsis, which will lead to multiple organ failure, the main cause of morbidity and mortality in burns (GOME and SERRA, 1999, p. 333).

Oxyhemodynamic monitoring now allows the clinician to continuously obtain cardiac output, right ventricular function, mixed venous blood oximetry and oxygen transport. The new pulmonary artery catheters instantly provide data on preload, cardiac contractility and afterload that were not previously available. This data is used to adjust cardiac output, which is defined by the adequacy of oxygen transport. The risk of catheter infection can be reduced by adequate asepsis and antisepsis when inserting and handling the catheter. Short-term use also reduces the risk of infection, since monitoring is often necessary in the initial phase of resuscitation (GOMES et al; 1995. p.192).

The aim of oxygen transport is to supply the cells with the oxygen they need to meet their metabolic needs at all times. If oxygen demand exceeds supply, progressive lactic acidosis will be present. The metabolism associated with lactic acidosis in very severe patients, such as those who have suffered extreme burns, is still poorly studied. Increases occur when mitochondria are unable to use pyruvate at the appropriate rate, either due to a deficiency in the cell's oxygen supply or excess demand, such as in excessive physical activity or catecholamine stimulation, and also due to a reduction in lactate clearance. Therefore, new studies need to be carried out to relate volume replacement in patients with severe burns to lactate levels (GOMES, 2001, p.151).

Any patient with more than 20% of their body area burned needs water support. A Ringer's lactate solution is infused to keep the patient's urine output between 30 and 50ml/h (GOMES and SERRA, 1999, p.333).

Over time, numerous formulas have emerged for the approximate calculation of fluids to be infused into the severely burned patient during the resuscitation phase. These formulas use crystalloid solutions, colloids or both, most of which are based on weight or body surface area and the percentage of burned area, all with the aim of trying to provide an ideal amount of fluid for adequate tissue perfusion (BOUNDY, 2004, p1014).

There is currently a consensus among various authors that the numerous formulas for replacement can only be used as a starting point, since replacement varies from patient to patient (GOMES and SERRA, 1999, p.333).

According to Moncrief, "blind adherence to a specific water formula and the rigid administration of volume in the regimens, despite variations in a patient's responses, lead to a poor outcome and a high mortality rate".

Modification of a given water replacement regimen should be made after appropriate clinical judgment and according to the patient's response.

The formulas can only be used as a starting point and roadmap by which adjustments and variations can and should be made.

The Parkland formula, devised by Baxter, is the most popular formula used worldwide. It recommends: 3 to 4ml of Ringer's lactate x kg x % SCQ.

This volume should be infused in the first 24 hours, and half the volume should be infused in the first 8 hours after the trauma (GOMES, 2001, p.151).

For resuscitation to be successful, it is extremely important to bear in mind that fluid therapy is a dynamic procedure par excellence, thus requiring permanent monitoring, especially in the first 24 to 48 hours after the burn (MARINI and WHEELER.1999p.1403-1419).

The Albert Einstein Hospital, in its intensive care unit, also recommends the above scheme (KNOBEL, 2006,P.360)

According to Gomes, the repositioning therapy for burns should be demystified, since it follows such simple principles, and yet many doctors are confused (TOCANTINS, 1988, p.40-56).

In his two-neuron theory, he states that only two neurons are needed to correctly reposition a burn patient. Once the hydrolytic solution to be used has been chosen, one neuron is enough to control the infusion drip and the other neuron to observe the urine flow in response to the infusion, i.e. volume replacement consists of a simple method whose objective is to maintain urine output between 30 and 50ml, and for children, around 1ml/kg/h (GOMES, 2001, p.151).

2.3.3 Trauma Associated Injuries

In the initial care of a major burn patient, it is important to look for signs or symptoms of associated trauma, often caused by fleeing the scene of the accident. Falls from great heights often occur in victims of electrical burns from high-voltage air networks and can cause bone fractures, head and spinal trauma. Pneumothorax, hemothorax, cardiac tamponade, chest fractures with unstable chest, and other traumas can also occur (HUDAK and GALLO, 1997, p.890-912).

A full head-to-toe examination should be conducted to determine any combined injuries. It is important that analgesia is only applied after this neurological assessment so as not to run the risk of applying a narcotic to a patient with neurological impairment (SMELTZER and BARE, 2002.p. 1434-1468).

2.3.4 Analgesia

Pain is a sensation that practically all burn patients experience and should be relieved after volume replacement has been started. Many other factors are also related to pain, such as associated trauma; the patient's psychological state; debris adhered to the burn such as tissue and tar; level of consciousness; previous use of alcohol or other drugs (TABORDA et al. 2004).

On admission, with the patient hypovolemic, the opioid can be administered intravenously, in small boluses, under the supervision of vital parameters. Intramuscular or subcutaneous use in this phase should be avoided because of the reduction in muscular and thermal blood flow due to hypovolemia, subsequently leading to the absorption of a large amount of the drug after the resuscitation phase, with the risk of respiratory depression, especially if repeated doses are used (GOMES, 2001, p.151).

We use the combination of midazolam and ketamine to debride, bathe and dress the patient, making it possible to handle the wound without discomfort for the patient. It is necessary to monitor the patient's heart rate and pulse oximetry (GOMES and SERRA, 1999, p.333).

2.3.5 Dressing

The treatment of the injury never takes precedence over the patient's life-threatening alterations, but it is an important aspect of care during the acute phase of the burn (GOMES et al; 1995. p.192).

Once the patient is hemodynamically stabilized, the dressing can be carried out under analgesia rather than anesthesia, when the burned area will be washed with running water and degermed with PVPI or chlorhexidine-based solutions for 8 minutes (GOMES, 2001, p.151).

After drying the area, an agent is applied topically, which can be 1% silver sulphadiazine, cerium sulphadiazine or even pure petroleum jelly. This is followed by an occlusive dressing using surgical compresses and crepe bandages applied in a slightly compressive manner (GOMES and SERRA, 1999, p.333).

Deep circular burns can act as "garrotes", not allowing vascularization of the extremities. Escharotomies are incisions in these deep burn areas, with the aim of decompressing them (unloading incisions). Generally, anesthesia is not required for the procedure, as the incised area is painless due to the burning of the nerve endings. It can also be performed on the chest to allow breathing movements (GOMES, 2001, p.151).

Another very important procedure is to take care with the patient's posture. In the case of burns to the face and extremities, the burned area should be kept elevated (30°) to reduce the formation of edema, which worsens tissue perfusion and deepens the injury (GOMES et al; 1995. p.192).

2.3.6 Tetanus prophylaxis

Extensive burns are considered wounds with a high risk of developing tetanus. Tetanus prophylaxis should be carried out in all burn patients, especially those with deep lesions with significant ischemic tissue involvement, without vaccination or incomplete or unknown vaccination (ATALLAH et al., 2004,p.668).

In patients who have never been vaccinated, are unaware of it or whose last booster dose was more than 10 years ago, start vaccinating with tetanus toxoid and prescribe anti-tetanus immunoglobulin at a dose of 250 to 500U IM or anti-tetanus serum (SAT) at a dose of 5,000 to 20,000U IM (GOMES and SERRA, 1999, p.333).

The preference for the use of immunoglobulin is due to the absence of acute allergic reactions and late immunological reactions frequently observed with the use of anti-tetanus serum (SAT). Even in the low-dose subcutaneous test that follows the application of SAT, allergic reactions can occur in sensitized people (GOMES, 2001, p.151).

Immunoglobulin is also indicated in patients infected with the human immunodeficiency virus, whatever their immunization history (SMELTZER and BARE, 2002, p.1432-1468).

Patients with humoral immune deficiency may not respond to the use of the toxoid, requiring passive immunization with immunoglobulin (GOMES, 2001, p.151).

2.3.7 Prophylaxis of Digestive Bleeding

Upper gastrointestinal bleeding caused by injury to the gastric mucosa is based on mucosal ischemia due to decreased perfusion induced by hypovolemia. Therefore, the initial prophylaxis is rapid and adequate volume resuscitation (GOMES, 2001, p.151).

Early feeding will also help to prevent this, by naturally raising gastric pH. The use of an enteral diet, administered drop by drop into the stomach via a nasogastric tube, will also raise the gastric pH without the risk of excessive alkalization of the stomach and subsequent bacterial colonization (GOMES and SERRA, 1999, p.333).

It is currently recommended to start the enteral diet in the first 6 hours after the trauma. The use of aluminum hydroxide, H2 blockers or proton pump blockers will be useful in critically ill patients who are unable to feed themselves and have not yet started an enteral diet (GOMES, 2001, p.151).

2.3.8 Initial Procedures Specific to Types of Burns

Depending on the type of burn suffered, specific precautions are required. Below is a list of burns and precautions, and summarized details can be seen in the table in ANNEX 4: Characteristics of the most common burns.

2.3.8.1 Electric burns

When an electric current passes through an individual, it can cause extensive internal damage. These injuries are extremely difficult to assess clinically in the initial phase and require frequent re-evaluation, as they often evolve as the injuries deepen, sometimes leading to the exposure of muscles, tendons and bones, as well as having significant clinical repercussions depending on the intensity, duration and characteristics of the agent to which the patient has been exposed. There can be serious damage to the deep tissues of a limb where the skin, except at the point of contact with the electric current, is intact (GOMES, 2001, p.151). The severity of electrical burns is linked to:

- Type of current (alternating current is more dangerous due to the greater risk of arrhythmias);
- Amount of current (the higher the amperage, the more serious the injury);
- Path of the current (it is not possible to know which path it is by looking only at the external lesions);
- Duration of contact (the longer the contact, the greater the severity) (MINISTÉRIO DA SAÙDE, 2002).

Electrical burns cause direct damage to the skin (entry and exit injuries) and arrhythmias, which are the most serious immediate injuries (ventricular fibrillation or asystole) (SOARES et al. 1996).

In pre-hospital care, professionals must:

. Self-protection.

- Assess the safety of the scene, if the victim is trapped in the power source, the first step is to turn off the power source before accessing the victim. Don't try to pull the victim away with pieces of wood or any other object.

. When the scene is safe, access the victim by approaching them as we have seen so far, as a trauma victim, performing the primary examination, being attentive to the signs of cardiorespiratory arrest due to possible arrhythmias, which is the most serious complication of electrical burns (ATALLAH et al., 2004,p.668).

. The victim should be monitored for cardiac function.

As it is not possible to determine the path and extent of the electrical burn, every electrical burn victim should be removed to hospital (SMELTZER and BARE, 2002, p.1432-1468).

Control of diuresis is extremely important in monitoring water replacement, since hydration is the vital support in the resuscitation of burn patients based on their pathophysiology. Diuresis control in large burn patients must be carried out rigorously using a long-term bladder catheter (HUDAK and GALLO, 1997, p.890-912).

Diuresis levels should be maintained at 30-50ml/hour in adults and lml/kg/hour in children. In the presence of hemoglobinuria or myoglobinuria, this monitoring should be stricter, as there is a risk of renal complications, and an attempt should be made to maintain levels above the recommended hourly diuresis. Diuresis should be maintained at 75-100ml/h in adults and 2ml/kg/h in children. From the fourth or fifth day after the burn, there may be an increase in diuresis due to the reabsorption of edema, which can lead to water overload (GOMES and SERRA, 1999, p.333).

The use of mannitol may be necessary. Metabolic acidosis is corrected with adequate perfusion and the addition of sodium bicarbonate to increase the solubility of myoglobin (PEREIRA, 2005).

A major concern is the effect on normal cardiac electrical activity. Serious arrhythmias can occur even after a stable cardiac rhythm has been achieved. Continuous cardiac monitoring is necessary for the first 24 hours after the injury. The limbs, when affected, almost always require scarotomies and fasciotomies to free vessels, nerves and swollen muscles confined to the fascial spaces. In the hands, special attention should be paid to the interosseous compartments

to prevent necrosis of the intrinsic muscles of the hand (ATALLAH et al., 2004,p.668).

2.3.8.2 Chemical burns

Similarly to electrical burns, the tendency of the assessor is to underestimate the appearance of the lesions in an initial approach. It is necessary to assess the extent and depth of the lesions at frequent intervals.

Chemicals can damage the skin and, when absorbed, also internal organs; in the case of inhalation, there can be serious damage to the respiratory system (GOMES and SERRA, 1999, p.333).

According to Gomes (2001, p.151), the severity of chemical burns is linked to:

- Type of substance;
- Concentration of the substance;
- Quantity of the substance;
- Duration of contact;
- Mechanism of action.

The victim is approached in the same way as any other trauma victim, paying attention to the following details:

- The professional providing the care must protect themselves from exposure by wearing suitable protective devices so that they don't get burned by the substance either;
- The clothes removed must be bagged and identified so that there is no tampering and no further accidents;
- If the substance is powdered, brush or wipe off the excess before irrigating the affected area;
- Try to identify the substance to make it easier to identify the antidote when necessary (MINISTÉRIO DA SAÙDE, 2002).

Acids, due to their pathophysiological mechanism, tend to stop the burn process around 48 to 72 hours after the accident, when patients generally stop reporting pain. Alkalis, with their high penetration capacity, tend to become chronic due to the difficulty in eliminating the agent, and the need for multiple escharotomies is common, as well as favoring infections due to the alkaline environment they establish (ATALLAH et al., 2004, p.668).

At the scene of the accident, it is advisable to remove all clothing and continue irrigation with water for 20 to 30 minutes. Chemical agents should be removed from the body surface immediately with running water. Delaying this measure allows tissue damage to continue. Powdered chemicals should be removed from the skin before washing the body surface area. No agent has been shown to be superior to water. Irrigation should be continued from the pre-hospital setting until the patient experiences a reduction in pain or burning in the wound (SMELTZER and BARE, 2002, p.1432-1468).

For eye burns, continuous irrigation with water or immersing the head in water tanks with open and close movements of the eyelids is recommended to remove the agent (ATALLAH et al., 2004,p.668).

Efforts to neutralize chemical agents are contraindicated due to a possible exothermic reaction, which will contribute to tissue destruction. Eye injuries caused by chemical substances also require continuous irrigation. Chemical burns are closely related to the work environment and predominantly affect young adults (GOMES, 2001, p.151).

2.3.8.3 Facial burn

They are considered serious injuries and usually require treatment in hospital. Due to the rich blood supply to the loose tissue, facial burns are associated with the formation of large edema, which can lead to significant changes in anatomical structures, with difficulty breathing and/or ingesting food (ATALLAH et al., 2004,p.668).

To minimize this edema formation, the patient's upper torso and head should be elevated to an angle of 30°. In children, elevating the head can reduce the potential for convulsions during resuscitation (GOMES and SERRA, 1999, p.333).

2.3.8.4 Eye burns

Eyeball involvement in the presence of a facial burn can be suspected if the patient reports blurred vision, has intense photophobia or the conjunctiva is hyperemic. Often, necrotic tissue forms on the ocular surface, which can appear as a black area on the conjunctiva or sclera, as well as a whitish membrane on the cornea (GOMES and SERRA, 1999, p.333).

If a burn to the globe is suspected, an ophthalmologist should be called as soon as possible. He will debride the necrotic areas or remove foreign bodies related to the burn, such as cigarette ashes, under typical anesthesia. The patient will then be observed daily until the eye wounds have healed (GOMES, 2001, p.151).

Clinical treatment generally includes the use of cycloplegic eye drops, antibiotic ointments, eye lubricants, therapeutic contact lenses or occlusive dressings and, in the most severe cases, topical corticosteroids. Corticosteroids should not be used for more than 14 days after the corneal burn to avoid limiting collagen production, impairing healing and increasing the risk of secondary infection. Topical beta-blocker drugs can also be instilled to lower intraocular pressure, if necessary (ATALLAH et al., 2004, p.668).

2.3.8.5 Hand and foot burns

These are areas of great functional importance and, like the extremities, are prone to greater circulatory impairment due to the small caliber of the vessels. The most important aspect of the physical assessment is to determine the vascular situation and the possible need for an escharotomy. The presence of a radial pulse does not include compartment syndrome. Monitoring digital and palmar pulses with an ultrasonic meter is the most accurate way of assessing tissue perfusion in the hand (GOMES and SERRA, 1999, p.333).

Elevate the extremity above the level of the heart to minimize the formation of edema. Moving the limbs involved for 5 minutes every hour will reduce edema. Dressings will only impair the ability to monitor circulation and should be avoided (GOMES, 2001, p.151).

2.3.8.6 Genital burning

There is a greater risk of contamination. Penile burns require the immediate insertion of a

Foley catheter to maintain the opening of the urethra (GOMES and SERRA, 1999, p.333).

2.3.8.7 Burned pregnant patient

The presence of pregnancy in a burned woman should be considered due to the complications that can occur for the mother and/or child. The possibility of pregnancy should be assumed in any woman of reproductive age (GOMES, 2001, p.151).

Flames and explosions are the most common mechanisms of burns. The outcome of pregnancy is determined by the extent of the burns to the pregnant woman. Spontaneous abortion can occur in patients with 60% or more of SCQ (GOMES et al., 1995, p.192).

After the above considerations have been taken into account, if there is a delay in freeing up space to treat the major burn patient in specialized units, the intensive care procedures listed in ANNEX 6 Nursing procedures in the acute phase should be initiated.

2.3.8.9 Complications of burns

Aggressive and rapidly initiated volume resuscitation has been an important gain in the survival of patients who have suffered major burns. With current pathophysiological and therapeutic knowledge, countless victims have survived hypovolemic shock and renal failure, which years ago caused the death of these patients, and are therefore exposed to the various complications inherent in the burn itself or resulting from the treatment (GOMES et al; 1995. p.192).

Mesenteric circulation is observed during hypovolemic shock. Complications that affect the major burn patient occur in the post-resuscitation period, such as hemorrhagic gastroduodenal lesions, acute pancreatitis, calculous cholecystitis, ischemic enteritis and bacterial translocation. Due to their importance, we will briefly recap the pathophysiology (GOMES, 2001, p.151).

Immediately after the thermal trauma, a significant decrease in mesenteric blood flow is observed, with a reduction in blood supply to the mucosa and submucosa of the jejunum, cecum and colon as early as five minutes after the trauma, with maximum dysfunction being observed around four hours later. A rapid recovery of flow occurs over the following 24 hours. With a slower recovery thereafter, flow abnormalities are observed up to around three weeks after the burn. The mechanisms that cause mucosal ischemia remain unclear, and the identification of mediators could facilitate the development of drugs or procedures that improve mesenteric blood flow, thus increasing survival in this group of patients (GOMES et al; 1995. p.192).

Studies carried out on burn patients show that even in those who are adequately resuscitated and maintain stable hemodynamic parameters, there is a significant reduction in mesenteric artery flow. Therefore, the altered hemodynamic state cannot be considered solely responsible for poor mesenteric perfusion. The renin-angiotensin system plays an important role in the pathophysiology of burns, with angiotensin II being an important vasoconstrictor agent acting on the mesenteric territory. The experimental use of angiotensin II receptor antagonists or angiotensin-converting enzyme inhibitors can prevent post-burn vasoconstriction, if used before causing burns in animal models (GOMES, 2001, p.151).

It is known that there is a physiological balance between the production of prostagladin I2 and thromboxane A2, and between nitric oxide and oxygen free radicals, which allows vascular tone to be maintained. When tissues are damaged by ischemia, the mechanisms controlling oxygen metabolism are compromised. The increase in the intracellular concentration of oxygen free radicals is capable of inactivating nitric oxide and can inhibit the production of prostacyclin by the endothelial cell and inhibit the production of prostacyclin by the endothelial cell and inhibit cyclooxygen synthases (COX-I and COX-II), without destroying TXA2 synthase. The final result of this process is a worsening of vasoconstriction (GOMES et al; 1995. p.192).

When an extensive area of skin is destroyed by a burn, a large amount of endotoxin-rich fluid produced in the under-skin region is absorbed and the patient's body loses control of the inflammatory process, which amplifies and develops a systemic reaction that is known as the systemic inflammatory response syndrome (SIRS), characterized by hyperthermia, leukocytosis with neutrophilia, tachycardia and tachypnea. It should be noted that this pro-inflammatory phenomenon is one side of the coin, the other being an anti-inflammatory response called the compensatory anti-inflammatory response syndrome (CARS). This theory was developed by the following observation: 1) many pro-inflammatory mediators, mainly interleukins 4, 10, 11 and 13, soluble TNF receptors and growth factor, can inhibit the immune response by decreasing the function of macrophages and B and T9 lymphocytes; 2) pro-inflammatory mediators can inhibit their own synthesis of natural antagonists; and 3) treatment with anti-inflammatory agents fails to control SIRS. These anti-inflammatory responses are physiologically used by the body to re-establish homeostasis and result in allergy, in these cases severe they increase susceptibility to infection in general. In patients with severe burns, after the resuscitation period, the inflammatory process calms down. They show a reduction in body temperature, heart and respiratory rates and the number of leukocytes fall, which can be related to CARS, increasing susceptibility to infection (GOMES, 2001, p.151).

In addition to these immunological alterations observed in SIRS/CARS of any etiology, patients who are victims of major burns have their own immunological deficiencies which greatly aggravate the infectious situation. Products from the burnt skin are absorbed and provide a large quantity of antigens that will be identified by macrophages, leading to the formation of suppressor cells. Many of the products of arachidonic acid metabolism, such as some prostaglandins and leukotrienes, act to decrease defenses by stimulating the production of suppressor T lymphocytes and increasing the suppressor activity of macrophages. There is also a decrease in complement levels, reducing the ability of phagocytic cells to chemotaxis, opsonization and phagocytosis. The production of immunoglobulins will also be reduced (GOMES et al; 1995. p.192).

2.3.10 Complications of the respiratory tract

2.3.10.1 Pneumonia

A common complication in patients who have suffered severe burns, airborne contamination occurs early and is related to several factors besides immune depression, such as bronchoaspiration, inhalation injury and the presence of a tracheostomy tube for mechanical ventilation. The clinical picture presented by the patient is one of deteriorating general condition, sustained high fever, cough and purulent expectoration. Radiographic examination shows bilateral diffuse pulmonary infiltrates. The treatment should be intensified bronchial flushing and the use of antibiotics specific to the infecting germ, and every effort should be made to identify it (ATALLAH et al., 2004,p.668).

Pneumonia can also be endogenous, caused by pathogenic microorganisms already present in the patient's flora when they are admitted. This form of infection was more common before the advent of topical antimicrobial therapy. Sources of hematogenous pneumonia include intestinal flora due to bacterial translocation, a contaminated burn area, suppurative thrombophlebitis, perforation of a hollow viscera, occult soft tissue infections and bacterial endocarditis. It can be prevented by avoiding the occurrence of infection in other sites by correcting hypovolemia, treating wounds with degermation, debridement and topical chemotherapy, and grafting deep wounds as quickly as possible . Veins, both superficial and deep, should also be punctured with strict asepsis and changed frequently, thus avoiding phlebitis. This form of pneumonia occurs later in life. An isolated pulmonary infiltrate is the most common early sign, which can later evolve into multiple infiltrates of random distribution that can form areas of extensive condensation that are difficult to differentiate from those of bronchopneumonia. Serial blood cultures should be carried out in order to identify the offending germ. Every effort should be made to detect and treat the primary focus (GOMES et al; 1995. p.192).

2.3.10.2 Pulmonary embolism

This is not a very common complication. The risk factors and prophylaxis for pulmonary embolism and deep vein thrombosis remain debatable. It is estimated in various published series that thromboembolic phenomena occur in between 0.4 and 7% of burn patients, although the burn is related to a state of hypercoagulability in its initial phase. Also predisposing factors to the occurrence of thromboembolic phenomena are the need for patients to remain in fixed positions for prolonged periods of time and the frequent need for surgery (GOMES, 2001, p.151).

Pulmonary thromboembolism has not been observed in several autopsy series. However, pulmonary microembolism has been observed with some frequency in major burn victims who die from infectious complications. In addition to infectious complications, risk factors for thromboembolism include lower limb burns, the advanced age of the patients, the extent of the burn and obesity. Thromboembolism prophylaxis should be instituted with the use of low-molecular-weight heparin only in these high-risk patients. Prophylaxis in all patients with low doses of unfractionated heparin is not part of the therapeutic routine, due to the risks of wound bleeding, thrombocytopenia and arterial thrombosis, which occur in 0.6 to 5% according to the literature (GOMES et al; 1995. p.192).

2.3.11 Urinary System Complications

2.3.11.1 Acute renal failure

It is defined as an abrupt drop in the glomerular filtration rate, and can be caused by changes in intra-renal hemodynamics, by an intrinsic disease of the renal parenchyma or by obstruction to urine flow (GOMES and SERRA, 1999, p.333).

With current knowledge of the pathophysiology and treatment of burns, mortality from hypovolemic shock and ARF has fallen sharply. Hypovolemic conditions are only observed in those patients who have delayed the start of treatment, either because of a delay in getting to a hospital or because of a delay in transfer to a specialized center, without hydration being started (ATALLAH et al., 2004,p.668).

Due to increased vascular permeability, the body loses around 4.4ml of fluid per kilogram per hour, thus requiring very aggressive and rapid fluid replacement. In the absence of adequate hydration, cardiac output and renal plasma flow are reduced, leading to ARF

(GOMES and SERRA, 1999, p.333).

Special treatment must be given to patients who have suffered electrical burns, charring or burns associated with crushing. These individuals can develop acute tubular necrosis due to the direct renal action of myoglobin degradation products released by the injured muscle. These patients require greater water replacement, often associated with osmotic diuretics, in order to promote a large urine output to eliminate the nephrotoxic pigments (GOMES, 2001, p.151).

Acute renal failure has currently been observed in patients who develop burn sepsis, forming part of the picture of multiple organ failure. This is the serious clinical condition that follows the infection of the burn that has not responded to the treatment instituted. This form is related to a higher mortality rate (GOMES et al; 1995. p.192).

Therefore, acute renal failure occurs in patients who are victims of severe burns, with a bi-phasic characteristic. It manifests itself between the first and seventh day, when it is secondary to hypovolemia or damage to tubular cells by myoglobin; and between the nineteenth and twenty-third day, when it complicates the burn infection (GOMES, 2001, p.151).

Another possible cause of kidney failure in burn patients is the use of nephrotoxic antibiotics, such as aminoglycosides and vancomycin, as well as amphotericin B, which is used to treat fungal infections. Loop diuretics can favor this complication (GOMES and SERRA, 1999, p.333).

The clinical picture of acute renal failure is characterized by a reduction in urine volume and a progressive increase in edema. As the disease progresses, other clinical changes can be observed: changes in mental state are frequent, and the patient can become disoriented, drowsy or torporous and evolve into a uremic coma; various gastrointestinal complications can occur such as digestive bleeding, anorexia, nausea, vomiting and ileus adynamicus. Laboratory tests show an increase in nitrogenous slags and a reduction in creatinine clearance. Electrolyte disturbances are common; the patient develops hypocalcemia, hyperphosphatemia, hypermagnesemia and hyperpotassemia, the latter being the electrolyte alteration that most leads to serious complications, such as muscle weakness and, above all, alterations in the conduction of electrical stimuli up to cardiac arrest (GOMES, 2001, p.151).

The prognosis for acute renal failure is very poor. This complication, when it develops, has a high mortality rate, even in large burn treatment centers. Studies show that until 1965 all patients with extensive burns who developed acute renal failure died, and although the mortality rate has decreased since then, the prognosis remains bleak, with a mortality rate of over 80% in adult patients. In children with burns, there was a drop in mortality due to acute renal failure from 100% between 1966 and 1983 to 56% between 1984 and 1997, with the reduction being related to adequate volume resuscitation, early excision of the burn and better treatment of the infection (GOMES and SERRA, 1999, p.333).

When the diagnosis of acute renal failure is made, conservative treatment should be instituted as soon as possible, with water and protein restriction and strict electrolyte control. When this treatment becomes insufficient to maintain homeostasis, dialysis treatment should be instituted. Nowadays, this therapy has been started earlier due to the need of the major burn patient for continuous water replacement, to maintain a high protein intake and due to the accentuated catabolism. Fixed values of urea, creatinine and potassium are no longer considered when starting the procedure, but it is more important to observe the rate at which slags rise, metabolic acidosis worsens and the clinical condition worsens (ATALLAH et al., 2004, p.668).

Peritoneal dialysis has not been used frequently due to the difficulty of installing and maintaining the catheter. The difficulty of installation is due to the fact that burns to the abdominal wall are common in patients who have suffered extensive burns. It is also difficult to keep the dialysis catheter free from contamination, and the risk of peritonitis is high. It can be less effective at removing both liquids and sludge, and is not indicated in septic and hypercatabolic patients. Intermittent hemodialysis is prolonged, for around 8-12 hours, with high flows and performed daily at least six times a week. The urea reduction rate is often greater than 65%. The new dialysis machines can be fully programmed, carrying out the necessary slag clearance and ultrafiltration, with less risk of hypovolemia and other complications. In addition to prolonged hemodialysis, continuous dialysis can also be indicated, which, strategically, can present difficulties in the treatment of burn patients, as frequent surgical procedures are required in these patients, as well as baths, dressings, physiotherapeutic exercises, etc (GOMES, 2001, p.151).

2.3.11.2 Urinary Tract Infections

It is a frequent complication due to the use of the indwelling bladder catheter used to control urine output in patients with severe burns. Other factors can contribute to infection, such as perineal burns, the use of broad-spectrum antibiotics, obstructive diseases of the genitourinary tract, etc (GOMES and SERRA, 1999, p.333).

In addition to these causes of ascending infection, the kidneys can also be the site of hematogenous infection from infectious foci located at a distance. The clinical picture is characterized by high fever, chills, dysuria and pain in the renal area. A urine test will show pyocytes, red blood cells and granular cylinders. Urine culture will confirm the infection and isolate the germ, providing the antibiogram. Empirical therapy should be started as soon as the urine is cultured and modified, or not, depending on the clinical response and the results of the examination. The most frequently isolated germs are Gram-negative rods, but Gram-positive cocci such as enterococci and fungi, especially Candida spp, can also be isolated (GOMES, 2001, p.151).

Infection prophylaxis is very important. The tube should be passed with the utmost care and asepsis, the urine collection system should be closed and the tube should be kept in place for as short a time as necessary, and it should be removed as soon as the patient's hemodynamic condition has stabilized (GOMES and SERRA, 1999, p.333).

2.3.12 Anemia

Due to the massive loss of water and tissue necrosis, we initially observe an increase in hemoglobin and hematocrit associated with an increase in free hemoglobin in the urine in patients who have suffered severe burns. Hemastocopy shows fragmented red cells and spherocytes, and intravascular hemolysis is confirmed by a drop in hepatoglobin levels and an increase in plasma metahemalbumin levels (ATALLAH et al., 2004, p.668).

With aggressive water resuscitation, there is a rapid drop in the concentration of hemoglobin and hematocrit, and significant anemia is usually present in the next few days after the burn (TOCANTINS, 1988, p.40-56).

Anemia is aggravated by the blood loss that occurs during procedures such as dressings, surgery and blood collection for laboratory tests, as well as the possibility of digestive bleeding (GOMES and SERRA, 1999, p.333).

The occurrence of a process of continuous hemolysis, as an aggravation of anemia, is controversial; some studies have shown few changes in the half-life of red blood cells in the post-burn period. Nor has a previously suspected bone marrow failure been confirmed (GOMES et al; 1995. p.192).

The use of recombinant human erythropoetin r-(HuEPO) in patients with extensive burns showed no statistically significant change in hematocrit, hemoglobin, reticulocytes, serum iron, ferritin, iron combining capacity and the need for transfusion compared to patients who did not use the medication. With burns, ferritin and erythropoietin levels increase, as does the reticulocyte count. The erythropoietin response to anemia appears to be largely intact, since there is an appropriate inversion between the degree of anemia and the magnitude of the entropoietic response (GOMES, 2001, p.151).

Anemia greatly aggravates the patient's clinical condition, and the replacement of concentrated red blood cells should not be delayed in critically ill patients who require surgery or have an associated infectious condition, and a hematocrit of over 30% should always be maintained (ATALLAH et al., 2004, p.668).

2.3.13 Gastrointestinal changes

2.3.13.1 ileo

Adynamic ileus is described as a complicating factor in burns in the first few hours after trauma. The classic picture of ileus is rarely observed, with abdominal distension, vomiting, nausea and absence of hydroaerial sounds on auscultation. Patients are more likely to vomit in the first few hours after the burn, mainly due to the large amount of water ingested before the start of hydroelectrolyte replacement, because of the intense thirst caused by dehydration. In the initial treatment of the patient, fasting should therefore be avoided and adequate hydration promoted (GOMES, 2001, p.151).

The treatment of infrequent cases of ileus is metoclopramide or bromopride to facilitate gastric emptying, restricting oral intake and delaying the start of enteral feeding. More serious cases may require the use of a nasogastric tube until gastric activity returns (GOMES et al; 1995. p.192).

2.3.13.2 Acute ulcers

The gastric and duodenal ulcers found in patients with severe burns are seen in the general hospital population and are generically called "stress ulcers" (SMELTZER and BARE, 2002, p.1432- 1468).

Acute gastroduodenal ulcer secondary to burns was first described by Swan in 1823. Curling, in 1842, described a case of duodenal ulcer in a major burn patient; although it was later shown that the lesions are more frequent in the stomach, and are often superficial, not penetrating the *muscularis mucosa, the* name - Curling's ulcer - became widespread (GOMES, 2001, p.151).

They affect all age groups, but are uncommon in patients with less than 20% of their body surface burnt, and their incidence is directly proportional to the surface burnt. They can occur as early as a few hours after the trauma, being more frequent in the second week after the burn and are commonly precipitated by the onset of sepsis. They are usually multiple, shallow, small (rarely exceeding 2.5cm), without an inflammatory halo around them and located in the stomach. They are rarely found isolated in the duodenum, unlike classic peptic ulcers. Acute duodenal ulcers, although less frequent, are the ones that bleed the most and can also perforate, requiring greater care. Bleeding is usually mild with spontaneous arrest; severe bleeding is a rare complication, with a reported incidence of 3%. Recent reports of massive bleeding requiring total gastrectomy are rare (GOMES et al; 1995. p.192).

Various mechanisms have been used to try to explain gastroduodenal mucosal damage. These include a reduction in the stomach's ability to protect itself, a reduced capacity for regeneration of the mucosa, ischemia of the mucosa, reducing the removal of hydrogen ion, a decrease in the bicarbonate buffer against hydrogen ion and the back-diffusion of acid (GOMES, 2001, p.151).

The patient rarely presents with symptoms of peptic disease, such as burning pain in the stomach. The diagnosis is usually made when upper gastrointestinal endoscopy is performed due to an episode of upper gastrointestinal bleeding (GOMES and SERRA, 1999, p.333).

We can prevent the occurrence of curling ulcers by using oral alkalizers, H-blockers such as cimetidine and ranitidine or proton pump blockers such as omeprazole and pantoprazole. As a routine, we discontinue these medications when using the enteral diet, which will provide excellent prophylaxis of mucosal damage and reduce the risk of bacterial colonization of the stomach, which can occur when the gastric pH rises. Colonization of the stomach of severely burned patients can lead to the transfer of bacteria through the stomach wall, causing distant infections (GOMES, 2001, p.151).

2.3.13.3 Esophagitis

It is mainly caused by the use of nasogastric or nasoenteral tubes, which facilitate the gastroesophageal reflux of acidic material. The patient complains of heartburn and retrosternal pain, aggravated by oral feeding (GOMES and SERRA, 1999, p.333).

Treatment is carried out by alkalizing the gastric environment, using drugs that facilitate gastric emptying, such as metoclopramide or bromopride, and keeping the patient in a sitting position, especially during postprandial periods. Occasionally it will be necessary to remove the nasogastric tube and suspend the enteral diet until the symptoms subside (GOMES et al; 1995. p.192).

2.3.13.4 Acute pancreatitis

Pancreatitis has been well documented for years in autopsies carried out on fatal victims of major burns, although it was not well recognized as a clinical complication of burn patients and currently, with the increase in survival of critically ill patients, this complication has been diagnosed (GOMES et al; 1995. p.192).

Patients develop elevated serum amylase and lipase levels which, when associated with a worsening clinical picture, are often related to the burn infection. They often present with a clinical picture suggestive of pancreatitis with spontaneous abdominal pain and pain on palpation, distension, vomiting and cessation of auscultation of hydroaerial sounds. They can develop into pseudocysts and abscesses (GOMES, 2001, p.151).

Risk factors include delayed hydration, insufficient resuscitation, burn sepsis, disseminated intravascular coagulation and inhalation injury, associated trauma and scarotomies. It can occur as a complication of a penetrating duodenal ulcer (NOVAES, 2003, p.56-61).

Conservative treatment consists of suspension of the enteral diet, use of a nasogastric tube for decompression, H blockers or proton pump blockers, analgesics, parenteral hydration and electrolyte replacement. The use of broad-spectrum antibiotics, including antipseudomonal drugs, should be started as soon as possible. With clinical, laboratory and imaging improvement, the nasogastric tube should be removed and the oral test diet restarted. When the evolution is unfavorable or the patient has a pancreatic abscess, surgery is mandatory, with a poor prognosis (GOMES, 2001, p.151).

2.3.13.5 Acute cholecystitis

It is an infrequent complication in burns patients and has two predisposing causes: firstly, the vesicle of organs compromised by a systemic infection; the second cause, probably the most common, is dehydration, associated with gastrointestinal and biliary stasis and hemolysis. The diagnosis is suspected when the burn patient is jaundiced, complaining of pain in the right hypochondrium, nausea, vomiting and abdominal distension. Ultrasound will reveal a distended gallbladder with thickened walls (GOMES, 2001, p.151).

Cholecystitis is therefore prevented by adequate hydration and early feeding. The treatment of this complication is surgical and as early as possible, in order to avoid perforation and biliary peritonitis. In very severe and unstable patients, percutaneous cholecystostomy, guided by ultrasound, can be performed with minimal risk to the patient (GOMES and SERRA, 1999, p.333).

2.3.13.6 Liver Lesions

In the first 24 hours after the burn, high serum levels of liver enzymes are observed in patients with severe burns, without any clinical manifestations. These changes tend to normalize within a few days and probably reflect a reduction in hepatic blood flow during the period of shock and resuscitation, mediated by inflammatory and vasoactive factors released at the time of the accident. Severe cases of liver necrosis have occasionally been reported (GOMES, 2001, p.151).

Late changes often accompany infection and hypoxia. Patients are jaundiced and laboratory tests show a predominance of right bilirubin and elevated alkaline phosphatase and gamma glutamyl transferase, characterizing a cholestatic pattern. Transaminases may also be slightly elevated. These alterations are characteristic of an unspecific and generalized inflammatory process and are associated with a bleak prognosis (GOMES et al; 1995. p.192).

Jaundice can also be aggravated by hemolysis secondary to infection and hemolytic reactions to transfused blood (GOMES and SERRA, 1999, p.333).

2.3.13.7 Superior Mesenteric Artery Syndrome

This is a rare disorder caused by the severe malnutrition to which major burns patients can be subjected if they are not adequately fed. Duodenal obstruction occurs due to the clamping of this organ by the superior mesenteric vessels, especially in individuals with asthenic complex who lose weight very quickly, leading to the loss of the fat pad that supports the mesenteric vessels (GOMES, 2001, p.151).

Treatment should initially be conservative, with gastric decompression and later re-feeding, adopting a posture and maneuvers that facilitate emptying. The most serious cases that don't respond to conservative treatment are submitted to surgery to perform a jejunostomy for feeding (GOMES et al; 1995. p.192).

2.3.13.8 Intestinal Injuries

Intestinal lesions are often not diagnosed clinically. They can occasionally be seen in severely ill patients, due to mucosal ischemia, which can cause ulcers of the small intestine or colon, which in turn can bleed or cause fecal peritonitis. The diagnosis can be suspected in patients who present with abdominal distension, food intolerance, vomiting and pain. The presence of intestinal bleeding makes it necessary to make a differential diagnosis with curling ulcer, a more common disease with the same etiological basis, which can also occur concomitantly. The bleeding site can be difficult to locate, occurring throughout the small intestine up to the rectum. Ischemic intestinal lesions are complications that occur more commonly in individuals with severe infectious conditions, which makes clinical diagnosis very difficult, but pathological examination, when carried out, detects a frequency of more than 50% of cases of ischemic intestinal disease in fatal burn victims. These complications are probably caused by the accentuation of the reduction in mesenteric blood flow, attributed to the vasoactive and inflammatory mediators released in the initial phase of the trauma (GOMES et al; 1995. p.192).

Increased intra-abdominal pressure can also be blamed for ischemia by increasing the pressure in the mesenteric and portal veins, impairing the flow through the mesenteric arteries; this increase in intra-abdominal pressure occurs due to increased capillary permeability, large volume replacement of crystalloids and hypoproteinemia, leading to edema of the intestinal loops and mesentery. There is the possibility that enteral nutrition, which brings so many benefits to these patients, contributes to ischemic bowel disease, due to the need for a large amount of hyperosmolar substance to be administered directly into the jejunum, which is compromised, causing greater metabolic stress and attracting a large amount of fluid into the lumen of the organ, thus increasing distension and reducing mucosal perfusion. Enteral nutrition can have adverse effects on the oxygen balance without it being possible for the body to increase the oxygen balance.

supply in the late stages of burns complicated by infection. These complications are prevented by rapid and adequate volume replacement, early feeding and probably by positioning the enteral feeding tube at the level of the stomach, when there is no risk of bronchoaspiration associated with drugs that facilitate gastric emptying. Surgical treatment is mandatory in cases of loop perforation and bleeding that is difficult to control (GOMES, 2001, p.151).

2.3.14 Cardiovascular complications

2.3.14.1 Acute Myocardial Infarction

Burn victims experience a state of hypermetabolism that is directly proportional to the extent of the burn. Hypermetabolism is evidenced by increases in oxygen consumption, cardiac output, minute ventilation and body temperature. This response is mediated by an increase in catecholamine levels. The myocardium, when stimulated by catecholamines, sharply increases oxygen consumption, and if the supply is not adequate to meet the demand, myocardial infarction can occur (GOMES et al; 1995. p.192).

This serious complication can evolve asymptomatically and not be recognized as a cause of shock and pulmonary edema in burn patients. Diagnosis and treatment do not differ from those of patients admitted to coronary units, with the exception of the use of fibrinolytics, which are contraindicated due to the risk of bleeding from the wounds (GOMES, 2001, p.151).

2.3.14.2 Cardiac Arrhythmia

It can be a complication of acute myocardial infarction or occur in isolation, and is the most frequent cardiovascular alteration seen in burn patients (NOVAES, 2003, p.56-61).

Electrical burns are an important cause of arrhythmia. When death occurs as a result of a low-voltage electric shock, it is due to the direct effect of the current on the myocardium, causing ventricular fibrillation. Cardiac asystole and respiratory arrest occur as a result of damage to the brain centers due to the passage of high-voltage current (ATALLAH et al., 2004, p.668).

Cardiac monitoring should be instituted in patients who are victims of electrical burns, since arrhythmias are common in these patients in the first few hours after the event. Extrasystoles, atrioventricular and intraventricular conduction disorders may occur. Treatment will be based on the type of arrhythmia, and various drugs and pacemakers may be used when indicated. Defibrillation at the time of the electrical accident would be indicated, but the availability of a defibrillator is rare, and can be replaced by the precordial blow applied firmly at the junction between the middle and lower thirds of the sternum (HUDAK and GALLO, 1997, p.890-912).

2.3.14.3 Phlebitis

This is an infection of the veins that are catheterized in the burn patient. It is directly related to the length of time the catheter remains in the lumen of the vessel. It can occur in both deep and superficial veins and is more frequent in the lower limbs (TOCANTINS, 1988, p.40-56).

Clinically, unspecific signs of infection are observed, such as high and persistent fever, chills, tachycardia and tachypnea. Pain to the touch over the puncture site is an early symptom of infection. Clinical data is therefore of low specificity. Only in more exuberant cases, at the site of puncture or venous dissection, can phlogistic signs and drainage of purulent secretion be observed. The initially localized disease is characterized by causing distant infections such as hematogenous pneumonia, pyelonephritis and bacterial endocarditis (GOMES, 2001, p.151).

All burn patients with an infection without an apparent focus should have their veins that are currently catheterized explored, as well as those that have already been punctured. The incisions should be opened, the vascular ligatures removed and the contents of the veins examined. The diagnosis is confirmed when the luminal contents are purulent. The treatment of this severe form called suppurative thrombophlebitis consists of excising the affected area of the vein involved, as well as the tributary veins that are macroscopically affected. Empirical systemic antibiotic therapy should be instituted, as already described, and the identification of the germ should be sought by carrying out blood cultures as well as a culture of the excised material (GOMES et al; 1995. p.192).

Probably because venipuncture is more difficult in children, there is a tendency for the catheter to remain in place for longer periods of time in these patients, and the risk of catheter-related infection and sepsis is more frequent in these patients (NOVAES, 2003, p. 56-61).

Prevention is achieved by frequently changing venous accesses in accordance with aseptic techniques, giving preference to the peripheral veins of the upper limbs (SMELTZER and BARE, 2002, p.1432-1468).

Dressings should be changed daily and the appearance of the puncture should be observed. Special attention should be paid to the ends of venous access multipliers (polyfix) that are not being used, to avoid them being left open and with residues of blood and medication inside, serving as a culture medium for the proliferation of bacteria (GOMES, 2001, p.151).

2.3.14.4 Infective Endocarditis

It has long been known that infection of the valves and tendon chordae occurs much more frequently in patients with severe burns than in the general hospital population. The primary foci of infection that serve as a source of cardiac involvement are located in the burn itself and in suppurative thrombophlebitis. The extent of the burn and the prolonged use of intravenous catheters are therefore risk factors for the development of infection. The likelihood of a burn patient developing endocarditis is proportional to the extent of the burn, but there have been reports of infection secondary to minor burns. The manipulation of wounds favors the occurrence of bacteremia. *Staphylococcus aureus* and Gram-negative bacilli are the most commonly isolated microorganisms in blood cultures (GOMES, 2001, p.151).

Often the presentation of endocarditis in burn victims is silent, with only persistent fever and positive blood cultures for the causative agent. In more exuberant cases, the diagnosis is suspected in those patients who present with general signs of infection, audible heart murmurs, cardiac arrhythmia or acute heart failure. Three carefully collected blood cultures are adequate to confirm the diagnosis in most cases (GOMES et al; 1995. p.192).

2.3.14.5 *Peripheral Arterial Insufficiency*

After a circumferential full thickness burn of an extremity, subdural edema can limit blood flow to the tissues. The extremity distal to the burn will show cyanosis, reduced capillary filling and neurological symptoms, especially paresthesia and pain. An ultrasonic flow assessment should be carried out, and if flow impairment is confirmed, an escharotomy should be performed (GOMES, 2001, p.151).

Patients with traumatic injuries associated with electrical burns or deep burns involving muscles may have edema below the muscle fascia which also leads to a reduction in arterial flow. In these cases, it is necessary to perform a fasciotomy (GOMES et al; 1995. p.192).

Occasionally, patients who are victims of high-voltage electrical burns and charring have all blood flow impeded to the affected limb. In these cases, an angiographic study is carried out and, if extensive arterial damage is confirmed, the area of gangrene is delimited and amputation is carried out, preferably flat, thus avoiding the development of an abscess in the stump (GOMES, 2001, p.151).

2.3.14.6 *Heart Failure*

Although difficult to diagnose clinically, cardiac dysfunction can be observed in the initial phase of treatment for patients with extensive burns; the data obtained from hemodynamic monitoring confirms the deficit. This reduction in cardiac output is not necessarily related to the loss of circulating plasma volume which occurs due to the large loss of liquids from the burn and increased capillary permeability in areas far from the injury. The mechanisms responsible for the cardiac deficit remain poorly understood and still controversial. A few years ago, some authors suggested the existence of circulating myocardial depressant factors released by the burned tissue. More recently, experimental studies have linked myocardial depression to pro-inflammatory cytokines such as tumor necrosis factor (TNF) and interleukin (IL) 1β, which are released in large quantities at the time of the accident. Further studies have linked the disorder to an increase in the production of nitric oxide by the inducible nitric oxide synthase (iNOS), due to the stimulation of inflammatory cytokines released by the burn. Nitric oxide, which is an endogenous vasodilator synthesized from L-arginine, when produced on a large scale, will have a damaging effect on vascular regulation and myocardial contractility (GOMES, 2001, p.151).

Clinically, heart failure is seen in severe patients, in the later stages, as part of multiple organ failure secondary to burn sepsis. In these cases, the diagnosis is established by the classic clinical alterations, such as generalized oedema, pleural effusion, tachycardia, bulbous rales, auscultation of the third heart sound, etc (GOMES et al; 1995. p.192).

2.3.14.7 Transfusion Complications

As a major burn patient requires large supplies of albumin, plasma, concentrated red blood cells, and possibly cryoconcentrates of clotting factors and platelets, they can become carriers of various infectious diseases transmitted by blood products and also be susceptible to hemolytic complications due to blood incompatibility (GOMES, 2001, p.151).

Hemolysis by alloantibodies can be intravascular and is commonly related to incompatibility in the ABO system. Symptoms include anxiety, tachycardia, tachypnea, flushing, chest or lumbar pain and nausea, followed by shock and signs of renal failure (GOMES et al; 1995. p.192).

Extravascular hemolysis is usually caused by antibodies of the Rh system, but other antibodies of the Kell, Duffy and Kidd systems also fit this pattern. The clinical manifestations are mild, usually malaise and fever, and relations are delayed. The best laboratory indicator is the increase in indirect bilirubin combined with the fact that the hematocrit does not reach the expected levels (GOMES, 2001, p.151).

There are many blood-borne infectious diseases, most of which, because they have a long incubation period, manifest themselves after discharge from hospital. These include AIDS, malaria, toxoplasmosis, brucellosis, syphilis, hepatitis, Chagas disease, cytomegalovirus, etc. Prophylaxis will be carried out through rigorous donor selection (GOMES and SERRA, 1999, p.333).

In addition to these diseases, blood can be contaminated by bacteria during handling or storage, leading to clinical changes ranging from fever and chills to bacteremic shock itself. Treatment consists of the suspension of blood, the use of antipyretics and promethazine and, in the case of shock, volume replacement and sympathomimetic amines; high doses of corticoids can be used in this case, and the blood used should be cultured in order to identify the contaminating pathogen (GOMES, 2001, p.151).

2.3.15 Imbalance of Preexisting Diseases

Various diseases can be complicated by burns. A state of hypermetabolism driven by the action of various hormones can be observed in patients with severe burns, which, combined with a large supply of saline, can decompensate both arterial hypertension and previously compensated heart failure. The same applies to endocrine diseases such as diabetes, adrenal insufficiency and hypothyroidism (GOMES, 2001, p.151).

Attention should also be paid to allergies, since the patient will usually use various substances orally, intravenously or topically that can lead to clinical manifestations of allergy, such as asthma or urticaria (GOMES and SERRA, 1999, p.333).

2.3.16 Toxic Shock Syndrome

This is a serious and rare disease caused by a superantigen (toxic shock syndrome toxin - TSST-1) produced by strains of *Staphylococcus aureus* that can contaminate burns, even small ones. Superantigens have the ability to induce a massive proliferation of T lymphocytes and the production of cytokines. It occurs more frequently in children than in adults, probably because they have a lack of specific antibodies to one or more toxins within the superantigen family. The initial symptoms occur in the first two to three days after the accident and are non-specific, with high fever, skin rash, tachycardia, tachypnea, vomiting, diarrhea and hypotension, which can evolve into shock and death (GOMES, 2001, p.151).

2.4 Systematization of Nursing Care for Burn Victims

In the process of Systematizing Nursing Care for patients suffering from thermal injury, the following stages are listed and described below:

2.4.1 Nursing history

In the Nursing History process, it is up to the nurse to assess the burn, following the following parameters: the extent and depth, as well as the time and circumstances surrounding it, and in the assessment analyze:

- The percentage of body surface burned;
- A depth of the burn;
- A anatomical location of the burn;
- If inhalation injury has occurred;
- A individual's age;
- A clinical history;
- Simutaneous lesions (SMELTZER and BARE, 2002, p.1432-1468)

It is also up to the nurse to assess the hemodynamic status, detect complications, infused and eliminated volumes as well as the response to pain and psychosocial disorders faced by the patient and family (SMELTZER and BARE, 2002, p.1432-1468).

2.4.2 Physical Examination

The physical examination is involved in the initial care examinations and complementary examinations carried out in the initial care of the major burn victim at the time of their rescue or care provided in the emergency units to which they are taken.

2.4.3 Diagnoses, interventions and expected results.

2.4.3.1 Resuscitation or acute phase of the burn;

Nursing diagnosis	Patient goals	Nursing interventions
Water volume deficiency: related to increased capillary permeability, capillary hydrostatic pressure, decreased osmotic colloid pressure, increased loss through evaporation.	The patient will maintain water balance and hydration.	**1. intake and excretion every 1 hour. Evaluate trends.** **2. Dose IV fluids to maintain urine output.** **3. Daily weight, vital signs every 1 hour.** **4. report urine output < 30 or> 70ml/h.** **5. monitorhematocrit and electrolytes every 12 hours as prescribed.** **6. Obtain urine samples and monitor as prescribed for hemachromagens, sugar or acetone.** **7. Monitor sensitivity every 1 hour.**
Impaired gas exchange: related to carbon monoxide intoxication and/or inhalation injury.	The patient will maintain adequate oxygenation.	**1. Assess and document breath sounds every 4 hours.** **2. administer humidified** O_2 **as prescribed.** **3. Monitor** O_2 **saturation with oximetry.** **4. Monitor carboxyhemoglobin levels as prescribed.**
	The patient will be able to mobilize lung secretions.	**1. Turn every 2 hours.** **2. coughing, deep breathing and spirometry encouraged every 1 hour.** **3. Suction every 1 to 2 hours.** **4. Assessing and documenting pulmonary secretions.** **5. Monitor** O_2 **saturation with oximetry, assess arterial blood gases as necessary.** **6. Assess for inhalation injury: scorched nasal hairs, burns around the mouth or neck, expectoration of soot, burns in a limited area.** **7. Monitor for indications of airway obstruction only: stridor, wheezing, extertors, hoarseness,** O_2 **desaturation.**

		8. Prepare for endotracheal intubation and mechanical ventilation, as prescribed.
Pain: related to burns, tissue damage.	The patient has a treatable level of discomfort.	**1. Explain the methods before and during the intervention.** **2. Assess the need for sedative agents.** **3. Assess the need for analgesia:** **verbalization, changes in vital signs and agitation.** **4. Use alternative methods of pain control, such as music and relaxation.** **5. Administer IV analgesia, as prescribed, before painful interventions and on assessment.** **6. Monitor and document the response to medication.**
High risk of injury: related to impaired tissue perfusion, response	The patient will have adequate arterial perfusion at all times.	**1. Remove tight clothing and jewelry.** **2. Monitor the extremities every hour for signs and symptoms of**
stress, immobility and loss of skin integrity.	extremities with circumferential burns.	**decreased blood flow: pulse oximeter, ultrasound blood flow detector every hour, color and temperature, capillary refill, presence of peripheral pulses.** **3. Raise the burnt extremities above the level of the heart.** **4. Stimulate extremity exercises for 5 minutes every hour.** **5. Prepare escharotomy or transfer to operating room for fasciotomy.**
	The patient will have no gastrointestinal bleeding.	**1. Measure and examine the drainage of the SNG.** **2. Measure the pH of the SNG drainage every 2 hours.** **3. Evaluate the pH pH.** **4. Report pH < 5.** **5. Administer antacids and histamine H2 receptor antagonists as prescribed by your doctor.**
	The patient's skin or uninjured tissues will remain intact.	**1. Pad the foot protector and the side bulkheads.** **2. Pad the compression areas.** **3. Protect the ears and nasal septum from compression by the TOT and SNG joints.**

		4. Perform active and passive movements every hour. 5. Apply immobilizations as necessary. 6. Apply lubricating ointments to the eyes every 2 hours.
High risk of infection: burn-related, impaired immune response,	The patient will be free of infection from the burns.	1. Cover the wounds with sterile sheets when transferring the patient. 2. Clean the wound according to the
invasive methods, immobility.		scheme: gently debride, trim the hair from the areas near the wound. 3. Cover the wound with topical antimicrobials as prescribed. 4. Administer tetanus toxoid prophylactically, as prescribed. 5. Use heating lamps to maintain body temperature. 6. Evaluate invasive route insertion sites twice a day. 7. Obtain sample, as prescribed, for culture and sensitivity and monitor the results. 8. Report heat spikes or increased leukometry.
Ineffective individual coping related to fear and anxiety, worry and forced dependence on health professionals.	Patients and their families have effective coping strategies.	1. Offer explanations in a reliable way. 2. Provide honest answers to questions. 3. Encouraging appropriate coping strategies: following the regular schedule of activities, rewarding positive behavior, allowing the patient as much control as possible over the treatment. 4. Prepare the family for the initial visit and accompany them to the bedside. 5. Provide emotional support during visiting hours. 6. Keep the family informed of the patient's condition on a daily basis. 7. Refer the family to the support services available.
impaired physical mobility related to burn edema, pain and joint contractures.	Achieving optimum physical mobility.	1. Position the patient carefully to avoid a flexed position in the burned areas. 2. Help the patient to sit up and walk early. 3. Request a physiotherapy assessment.

		4. Use splints and exercise equipment recommended by the therapist. 5. Encourage self-care to the limit of the patient's ability.

2.4.4 Nursing evolution

In the process of evolution we can observe the following results in specialized treatment institutions if the interventions applied in the outpatient units of the industries and/or plants have been applied properly:

1. Achieve optimum water balance

a) Maintains intake, output and body weight that correlate with the expected pattern.

b) Vital signs and central venous and pulmonary arterial pressures within expected limits.

c) Demonstrates increased urine output in response to diuretic or vasoactive drugs.

d) He has a heart rate of less than 110 bpm in normal sinus rhythm.

2. No localized or systemic infections.

a) Presents lesion culture results showing minimal bacteria

b) Normal urine and sputum culture results.

3. Demonstrates anabolic nutritional status.

a) Gains weight daily after initial loss due to hydric diuresis and oral intake of food or liquid.

b) It shows no signs of protein, vitamin or mineral deficiency.

c) Fully satisfies nutritional needs through oral intake.

d) Participates in the selection of a diet containing the prescribed nutrients

4. Demonstrates improved skin integrity.

a) It generally supports intact skin that remains free from infection, pressure and injury.

b) They show the remaining areas of exposed lesion that are pink, re-epithelialized and free of infection.

c) It shows graft donor sites that are clean and healed.

d) It shows healed lesions, which are soft and smooth.

e) It shows that the skin is lubricated and elastic

5. It shows minimal pain.

a) Requests painkillers only for specific procedures to care for the injury or for physiotherapy activities.

b) He reports minimal pain.

c) It does not provide physiological or non-verbal indications that the pain is moderate or severe.

d) Use pain control measures such as nitrous oxide, relaxation and distraction techniques to deal with and relieve discomfort.

e) You can sleep without being disturbed by pain.

f) She reports that her skin is comfortable, with no itching or feeling of retraction.

6. Shows great physical mobility.

a) a. Improves joint range of motion on a daily basis.

b) Demonstrates pre-injury range of motion in all joints.

c) There are no signs of calcification around the joints.

d) Participates in activities of daily living.

7. Use appropriate coping strategies to deal with problems after burns.

a) Verbalizes reactions to burns, therapeutic procedures and losses.

b) Identifies the acceptance strategies used effectively in previous stressful situations.

c) Accepts dependence on health professionals during the acute phase.

d) It expresses a realistic view of the problems arising from the burn and plans for the future.

e) Cooperates with health professionals in the necessary therapy.

f) Participates in decision-making regarding treatment.

g) It resolves the grief over the losses caused by the burn.

h) Set realistic goals for plastic surgery and results.

8. Relates appropriately in patient/family processes.

a) The patient and family verbalize their feelings about the change in family interactions.

b) The family supports the patient emotionally during hospitalization.

c) The family claims that their needs are met.

9. No complications.

a) Clear lungs on auscultation.

b) He has no dyspnea or orthopnea and can breathe easily when standing, sitting or lying down.

c) Normal heartbeat with no signs of jugular stasis.

d) They experience urine output, central venous and pulmonary arterial pressures, and cardiac output within normal limits.

e) Normal blood, sputum and urine culture results.

f) Maintains arterial blood gas values within normal limits.

g) Normal lung compliance.

h) No damage to bladder organs.

i) He has a stable heart rhythm (SMELTZER and BARE, 2002, p.1432-1468).

3 DISCUSSION

3.1 Table 1: Burns update protocols for occupational nurses.

Subjects Authors	*Burns and polytrauma*	*Service Protocols*	*Burned area surface*	*Indication of hospitalization*	*Volume replacement*	*Nursing Care*
Atallah, Cega, Schiavon, Kikuchi and Cavallazzi, 2004.	It specifies that every burn victim is a polytraumatized person and should be treated as such.	Safe place, Stop contact with the damaging agent, start A B C D Efollow the treatment: cooling, debridement, treatment of the burned area, analgesia, volume replacement.	It doesn't specify.	It doesn't specify.	2 to 4 ml of lactated Ringer's solution / body weight / % of the burn surface (Brooke's formula).	It doesn't specify.
Flavio Novaes, 2003	The approach should always be made on an emergency basis and most of the time in generalist institutions that are not specific to treating this type of occurrence.	Take a careful history of the patient, check the airways, pulse oximetry and RR, blood perfusion with S/N escharotomy and check for polytrauma, after checking the burn area and volume repositioning.	It specifies the Rule of Nine, but emphasizes the Lund Browder Diagram.	Lesion 3° >5% SCQ. Lesion 2° >20% SCQ. Burns to the face, hands and feet, perineum and genitals, circulatory impairment, electrical or chemical discharges or those associated with trauma. People with CHF, SAH, DM and self-immolation.	It suggests the Parkland Scheme.	It doesn't specify.
Gomes, Serra, Guimaraes, 2001	It doesn't.	Assessment of respiratory failure, venous access, analgesia, stopping the heat source and cooling the patient, anamnesis, and determining SCQ.	Rule of Nines in adults but emphasizesthe Lund Browder Diagram.	Lesion 3° >10% SCQ. Lesion 2° > 20% SCQ in adults and 10% in children. Burns to the face, hands, feet, genitals, extremities, interfering with circulation. Electrical burns, associated with trauma and smoke poisoning.	He suggests infusing a crystalloid solution in the proportion of 2 to 4 ml/kg/% of the SCQ (adaptation of Brooke's formula).	It doesn't specify.
Hudak and Gallo, 1997	It doesn't.	Safe place, remove jewelry and tight clothing, venous access, SNG, airways, oxygen therapy, administration of tetanus toxoid, warming the patient	The rule of nine is most commonly used for adults and the Land Browder method for infants and children.	It doesn't specify.	Baxter's or Parkland's formula.	It specifies six nursing diagnoses containing 57 interventions respectively.

		to avoid hypothermia, monitoring and water resuscitation.				
National Safety Council, 2002	It doesn't.	Stop contact with the damaging agent, evaluate the ABC, assess the depth of the burn and its extent.	Use the rule of nine.	It doesn't specify.	It doesn't specify.	It doesn't specify.
Smeltzer and Bare, 2002	It doesn't.	Stop contact with the damaging agent, Apply A B C D E F (F being fluid resuscitation).	It uses the Rule of Nine in the pre-hospital unit, the Lund and Browder Method in emergency units and the Palm Method as an option in care.	It doesn't specify.	2 to 4 ml Ringer's lactate / weight body/ % of burn surface (Brooke's formula).	It specifies ten nursing diagnoses containing 69 interventions respectively.
Soares, Almeida, Gonçalves, 1996	It doesn't.	Stop contact with the harmful agent, airway approach with oxygen therapy and hemodynamic approach with volume replacement.	Use the rule of nine.	It doesn't specify.	2 to 4 ml electrolyte solution/ body weight/ % of burn surface.	Alista only interventions.
Taborda, 2004	It relates burns as a systemic trauma and not just skin lesions.	It recommends AB CDE followed by anamnesis and SCQ calculation.	The rule of nine is most commonly used for adults and the Land Browder method for infants and children.	Table: Triage of Burn Victim Patients, cited in Annex 3.	4 ml Lactated Ringer's solution / body weight/ % of burn surface (Brooke's formula)	It doesn't specify.
Tocantins, Gomes, 1988	It doesn't.	It does not specify emergency care.	It uses the Lund Browder Diagram.	It doesn't specify, the article deals with patients already hospitalized.	It suggests and follows the Parkland and Baxter scheme.	It doesn't specify.
Soares, 1998	It doesn't.	It establishes the priority of airway and oxygen therapy, venous access monitoring, infection prophylaxis, analgesia, avoiding hypothermia, laboratory tests and radiodiagnostics.	It suggests a rule of Nine.	It doesn't specify.	He does not suggest but lists the following schemes: Parkland and Baxter, Evans, Brooke, hypertonic saline and the consensus formula.	It lists 20 nursing interventions, which are more like the specific functions that nurses must carry out when providing care.
	The major burn victim can be a	Secondary care, intensive care	Does not specify	It has a table listing the severity and	Does not specify	List 55 nursing actions to be

	victim of polytrauma, sothe use of the usual trauma assessment is required			whether hospitalization is indicated		carried out in the acute phase
Santos, 2007	Listed as the fourth leading cause death by trauma	It addresses care for the type of burn and the moment of service	It suggests the Rule of Nine.	It only indicates a hospitalization.	It doesn't mention it.	List some of the interventions to be carried out during the service.

Flavio Novaes(2003), coordinator of the burns treatment unit at Santa Casa de Limeira, states that there is an increasing concept that the first care given to a patient can directly determine its evolution, which is why the approach should always be carried out on an emergency basis and most of the time in institutions with a generalist nature and not specific to the treatment of this type of occurrence, which implies that every burn is a polytrauma, Taborda (2004) points out that burn patients don't just have skin lesions, while Atallah, Higa, Schiavon, Kikuchi and Cavallazzi (2004) in their book Emergency Medicine Guides emphasize that burn patients are polytraumas and should be treated as such. The other six authors listed don't even relate burns to polytrauma. Recently, Elias Knobel (2006) and the author Nivea Cristina Moreira Santos (2007), in their work, point out that the major burn victim can be a victim of polytrauma, so the use of the usual trauma assessment is required.

In view of these considerations, it was observed that the effectiveness of initial care for major burns depends on a complete assessment of the patient, not only taking into account the injuries that are visible and external, but which may contain a major internal trauma, an injury that can cause irreversible damage if not treated correctly, such as cardiac arrhythmias, abdominal or cervical trauma.

Among the protocols for the care of major burn victims, the National Safety Council (2002) specifies the initial care according to the type of burn suffered by the patient, with each type of burn adopting a specific approach, while the authors Tocantins-Gomes (1988) and Knobel (2006) do not even list an initial procedure, The other authors listed in the table above suggest interrupting the thermal injury and starting the ABCDE, the same applied to polytraumatized patients, with emphasis on the burn suffered by the patient, examining and evaluating the burn areas, such as calculating the burned body surface area and the degree of burn.

Hudak-Gallo (1997), Knobel (2006) and Soares also emphasize the of tetanus toxoid as a prophylaxis against tetanus during initial care. Elias Knobel(2006) lists secondary treatment in intensive care units.

When it comes to initial care for a major burn victim, we need to describe the techniques, how it is carried out and the essential steps to be taken in order to provide effective help to the patient. Among the ways mentioned, it was observed that first of all, the victim should be moved away from the heat source, and then the care applied to the polytraumatized should be provided, following the ATLS, as listed below:

1. Remove the patient from the heat source;

2. "See, hear and feel" to see the expansion of the chest, hear the sounds of breathing and feel the exhaled air, so that the airways can be cleared, with control of the cervical spine;

3. Ventilation, providing oxygenation to the patient, either by mouth-to-mouth breathing during on-site care or by O_2 masks and catheters;

4. Circulation, checking the heartbeat with CPR in case of CPR, paying attention to possible open traumas where there is bleeding, which should be compressed to minimize blood loss and provide venous access for volume replacement.

5. In this phase we observe the level of consciousness, assessing how well the person responds to questions and stimuli.

6. Finally, a complete physical examination should be carried out, assessing the depth of the burn, its extent and observing signs of soot in the nostrils and mouth, which can signal respiratory complications.

7. after these measures, immobilization and removal to emergency units or a specialized hospital.

Another subject to be taken into consideration and of fundamental importance is the calculation of the burned body surface area. The authors Atallah, Higa, Schiavon, Kikuchi, Cavallazzi(2004) and Knobel(2006) mention the SCQ for calculating volume replacement, but do not suggest any way of doing this calculation; The authors of the National Safety Council (2002), Soares - Almeida - Gonçalves (1996), Soares (1998) and Santos - Nivea (2007) only suggest the Rule of Nine as being easy to interpret in emergency units, which contradicts Novaes(2003), Gomes - Serra - Guimarâes(2001), Smeltzer - Bare,(2002) and Taborda(2004), who suggest the Rule of Nine for adults and the Lund Browder Diagram for infants and children. Novaes points out that due to its ease of application, the rule of nine is suggested for urgent or emergency care, while the Lund Browder diagram is preferred in specialized services, due to its characteristic of more adequately fractionating the burn segments and taking age variations into account. Only the authors Tocantins - Gomes (1988) adopted the Lund Browder diagram.

As a fundamental part of care, the calculation of the burnt body surface must be as accurate as possible, as this determines the patient's fate as well as the treatment and blood volume to be used.

And when talking about SCQ, we have the Indication for Hospitalization through this calculation, and the authors Atallah - Higa - Schiavon - Kikuchi - Cavallazzi(2004), Hudak - Gallo(1997), National Safety Council(2002), Smeltzer - Bare(2002), Soares - Almeida - Gonçalves(1996), Tocantins - Gomes(1988) and Soares, Edina(1998) disregard the fact that the burn patient requires hospitalization for specialized treatment, and a suitable way of assessing this is suggested by Taborda (2004) and listed in Annex 3. Elias Knobel (2006) also specifies, using a table, classifications that suggest treatment, whether outpatient or inpatient, for burns, but it is not as precise and detailed as the one suggested by Taborda (2004).

Another issue to take into consideration is volume replacement. The authors Atallah - Higa - Schiavon - Kikuchi - Cavallazzi(2004), Gomes - Serra - Guimarâes(2001) and Taborda(2004), adopt the replacement factor, suggesting the infusion of crystalloid in the proportion of 2 to 4 ml/kg/% of the surface area of the burned area, The total volume of liquids to be infused is determined over the course of treatment, stressing that 2/3 of this volume should be infused in the first eight hours after the trauma, according to Brooke's scheme, while Novaes(2003), Hudak - Gallo(1997) and Tocantins - Gomes(1988) adopt the Baxter and Parkland scheme, Tocantins (1988) justifies this by saying that Baxter demonstrated a similar behavior between crystalloids and colloids in the first 24 hours after the burn, and that crystalloids result in lesser effects in the medium term, such as sequestration of protein elements in the interstitial space, and greater ease of rescue when vascular alterations return. Knobel(2006) and Santos(2007), however, make no mention of how to restore blood volume in these patients. Although Knobel(2006) deals with intensive care unit issues, this is a very important detail that is overlooked by the author and his collaborators.

However, the assessment of the burn surface, the care protocols, the indications for hospitalization and volume replacement would only be successful with effective nursing care, and of the eleven authors listed above, only four mention the Systematization of Nursing Care, with Hudak - Gallo (1997) and Smeltzer - Bare (2002), mention diagnoses, interventions and recovery goals, while Soares, Edina(1998) only lists twenty nursing interventions that are more like the initial care that should be provided at the time of treatment, without specifying diagnoses. Soares, Almeida and Gonçalves(1996) only list interventions such as: Interrupt contact with the aggressor; remove clothing that is not adhered; remove jewelry and ornaments; ensure a patent airway, protecting the cervical spine; provide oxygen therapy 12 to 15 l/min by mask; provide peripheral venous access with a large-caliber vein and take blood samples for typing, Hb, Ht, CBC, electrolyte dosage; monitor the patient; protect burned areas with a sterile cover; perform bladder catheterization and control urine output; prepare equipment and materials for advanced life support and be prepared to start resuscitation maneuvers, if necessary.

Knobel (2006) in his book written with 66 nurses, mentions 55 nursing actions to be carried out in the acute phase without mentioning any nursing diagnosis.

With accurate diagnoses and interventions, the patient's evolution after emergency treatment, together with the appropriate medical procedures, results in a faster and less traumatic recovery for the patient.

Although not mentioned above in the effective volume replacement, there is a good urine output, and in this regard, the authors Novaes (2003), Knobel (2006), Gomes - Serra (1999), Tocantins - Gomes (1988) consider that among all the methods of hemodynamic monitoring during the resuscitation of the burned patient, the urine output is the best of all. To this end, the method routinely indicated in adults with a burn area of more than 30%, the desired output is 30 to 50 ml/h or 1ml/kg/hour for children, reflecting minimum renal perfusion.

The authors Hudak - Gallo(1997), Soares(1998), Santos(2007) and Smeltzer - Bare(2002) do not mention the importance of urine output in the assessment of hemodynamic status, but both authors list nursing interventions requesting urine output control.

Effective control of urine output in burn patients is extremely valuable, as it helps to measure how hemodynamically stable the patient is.

4 FINAL CONSIDERATIONS

A burn of any size can be a serious injury, and first aid nurses must be able to assess injuries quickly and develop a treatment plan based on priorities.

The initial therapy strategy is based on the type, extent and degree of the burn, as well as the resources available. Bear in mind that treating the injury never takes precedence over life-threatening injuries.

Remember that the onset of symptoms associated with all types of inhalation injury is so unpredictable that the patient must be observed rigorously, and that any patient with the possibility of inhalation injury should immediately receive 100% humid oxygen through a mask.

Nurses should be aware that the aim of volume replacement is to maintain vital organ functions while controlling the complications of inadequate therapy. Excessive volumes of repositioning fluid can increase the formation of edema, causing a decrease in tissue oxygen tension and greater ischemic aggression in injured cells, potentiating tissue damage and increasing the risk of infection.

Also a complication of hyperhydration is pulmonary insufficiency resulting from both a reduction in chest wall compliance due to tissue edema and an increase in blood volume during edema mobilization.

Underhydration maintaining hypovolemia can prolong the state of shock, exacerbate metabolic acidosis and induce renal failure. It can also contribute to tissue ischemia, a condition capable of aggravating the level of suffering in the injured areas, thus producing areas vulnerable to infectious complications.

We know that there is still no consensus on the quantity and composition of fluids to be given during this period, but it is undeniably important for the patient's survival that this volume replacement is adequate and starts early.

Nurses must also be prepared to know how to transfer a major burn patient to a specialized center.

Volume replacement should be instituted as soon as possible, preferably before the patient arrives at the hospital. Delayed resuscitation leads to high mortality, not only because of the development of hypovolemic shock, renal failure and metabolic acidosis, which would be the terminal complications of a patient who has been without hydration for hours, but mainly because of altered gastrointestinal perfusion.

But for effective care, the Systematization of Nursing Care in all its forms, the nurse's knowledge of the burn, the pathophysiology, the rules of approach guarantee the effectiveness of the patient's treatment and recovery.

5 BIBLIOGRAPHICAL REFERENCES

American Heart Association, Paiva E . **SAVC Manual for Providers**. Rio de Janeiro, 2002 - handout.

-Atallah AN, Higa SEM, Schiavon LL, Kikuchi LOO, Cavallazzi RS. **Guide to Emergency Medicine**. Barueri: Manole; 2004. 668p.

-Boundy J, transl. Cosendy CH. **Medical and Surgical Nursing**. Rio de Janeiro: Reichmann & Affonso; 2004.1014 p.

- Carmen HS. **Burns.** [Accessed 12/10/2006] available at http://www.ufrrj.br/institutos/it/de/acidentes/queima.htm

- **Dicionârio de Administraçâo** de **Medicamentos na Enfermagem** 20032004, Rio de Janeiro: EPUB; 2002.

- Gomes DR, Serra MCVF, Guimaraes jr. LM. **Current Conducts in Burns**. 1st ed. Rio de Janeiro: Revinter; 2001.151p.

- Gomes DR, Serra MCVF, Pellon MA**. Burns**. Rio de Janeiro: Revinter; 1995. 192p.

- Gomes DR, Serra MCVF. **The Burned Child**. Rio de Janeiro: Eventos;1999. 333p.

- Hudak CM, Gallo BM. **Intensive Nursing Care**. A Holistic Approach, Rio de Janeiro: Guanabara Koogan; 1997. 912p.

- Johnson M, Bulechek G, Dochterman JM, Maas M, Moorhead S. **Nursing Diagnoses, Outcomes and Interventions - Linking NANDA, NOC and NIC**. Porto Alegre: Artmed; 2005. 506p.

- Kawamoto EE, Fortes JI. **Fundamentals of Nursing**. rev. and ampl. Sao Paulo: EPU; 1997. 248p.

- Knobel E. **Care of the critically ill patient**. Sao Paulo: Atheneu; 2006. 360p.

- Marini JJ, Wheeler AP. **Intensive Care**. Sao Paulo: Malote; 1999. 1419p.

- Ministry of Health. **Emergency Unit Protocols**. 10th ed. Brasilia, 2002 - handout.

- Moraes, MVG. **Occupational nursing: programs, procedures and techniques**. 3° Ed.rev. São Paulo: làtria, 2009, 190p.

- National Safety Council, trad: Fonseca E. **First Aid**. 4th ed. Sao Paulo; 2000. 248p.

-North American Nursing Associstion, transl. Correia C. **NANDA Nursing Diagnoses: Definitions and Classification** - 2003-2004. Porto Alegre: Artmed; 2005. 300p.

-Novaes FN. **First Aid to the Burned Patient**. Brazilian Journal of Medicine. 2003; 84 (5): 61p.

-Pereira LC. **Drugs and Solutions Used in Emergencies**. São Paulo, 2005 - handout.

-Santos, NCM. **Urgência e emergência para a enfermagem: do atendimento pré-hospitalar APH à sala de emergência**. 4ª ed.rev. e ampl.São Paulo: làtria, 2007. 167p.

-Sassine SW, Moura DF Jr, Laselva CR. Burns. In: Knobel E. **Terapia Intensiva - Enfermagem**. São Paulo: Atheneu; 2006. 2490p.

-Secretaria da Saùde do RJ. [Accessed 12/10/2006] available at http://www.saude.rj.gov.br/Queimaduras/classificacao.shtml

-Bauru Union of Employees in Health Services Establishments. **Basic Course in Urgencies and Emergencies** - Emergency Room. Bauru, 1999 - handout.

-Cruz ICF, Cabral IE, Figueiredo JEF, Lisboa MTL. **Tratado de Enfermagem Médico-Cirùrgica**. 9th ed. Rio de Janeiro: Guanabara Koogan; 2002. 1468p.

-Soares E. Emergency Department. **First Aid to Patients with Burns: Nursing Intervention**. Revista de Enfermagem da UERJ.1998; 6 (1): 251p.

-Soares LMCA, Almeida RP, Gonçalves VCS. **Manual for the Advanced Emergency Care Course for Nurses**. Sao Paulo, State Health Department; 1996 - handout.

-Taborda AC, Frison AA, Diarcadia ALS, Palhares AAN, Duarte AR, Ferreira DJ, et.al. **Advanced Urgent and Emergency Care Course**.Sao Paulo; 2004 - handout.

-Tocantins R, Gomes DR. **Burns**. Brazilian Journal of Medicine. 1988; 56p.

6 ANNEXES

6.1. ANNEX 1: Post-burn physiological changes

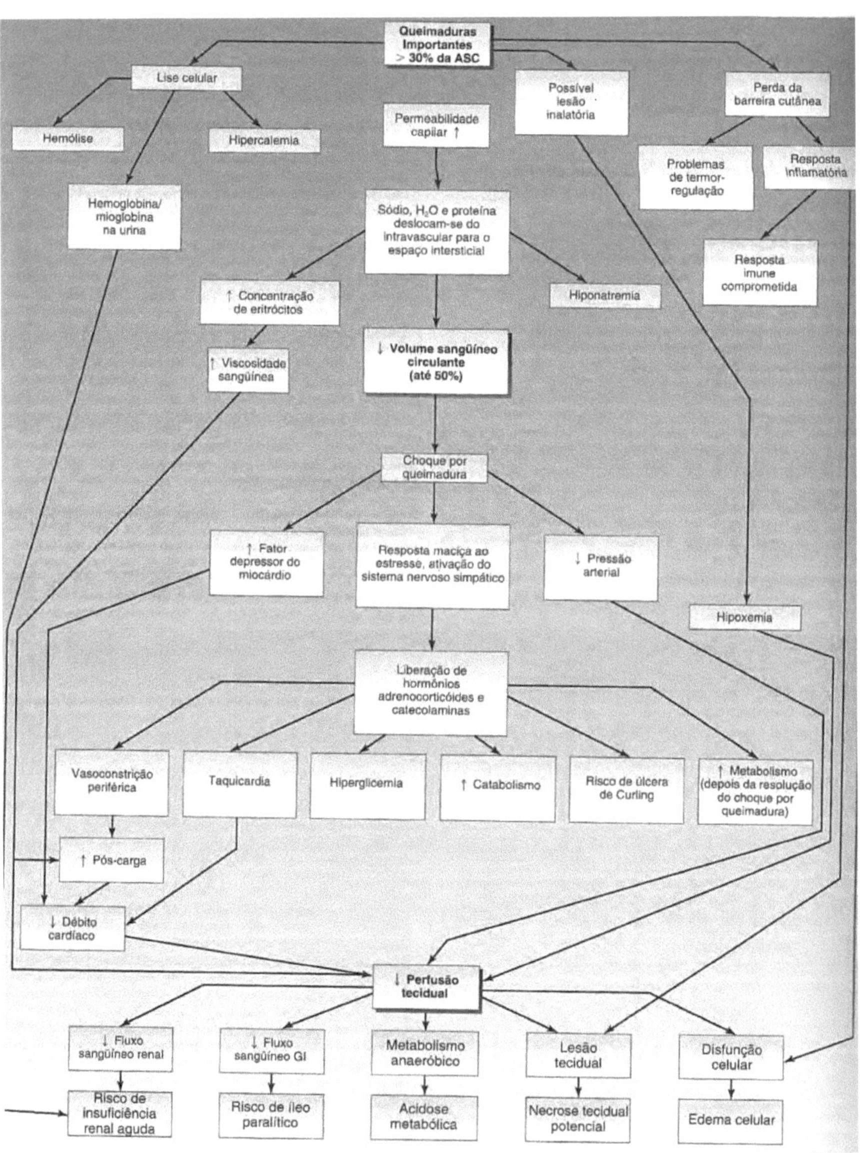

Source: SMELTZER, Suzanne C; BARE, Brenda G. trad. Isabel Cristina Fonseca da Cruz, Ivone Evangelista Cabral, José Eduardo Ferreira de Figueiredo e Márcia Tereza Luz Lisboa - Tratado de Enfermagem Médico-Cirùrgica, 9° ed.

6.2. ANNEX 2: Fluid Replenishment/Reanimation Formulas

First 24 hours				Mondays 24 Hours		
	Electrolytes	**Colloid**	**Glucose in water**	**Electrolytes**	**Colloid**	**Glucose in water**
F.D. Moore's recipe for burns.	1,000 - 4,000 ml of lactated Ringer's solution and 1,200 ml of saline solution 0,5N	7.5% body weight	1,500 - 5,000ml	1,000 - 4,000 ml of lactated Ringer's solution and 1,200 ml of 0.5N saline solution	2.5 % of body weight	**1,500 - 5,000 ml**
Evans	Normal saline solution, 1 ml/Kg/% of the burn.	1.0 ml/Kg/% of burn	2,000 ml	Half of the first 24 hours required	Demands of the first half hour	**2,000 ml**
Brooke	Lactated Ringer's 1.5 ml/Kg/% of the burn	0.5 ml/Kg/% of burn	2,000 ml	Half to three-quarters of the demands of the first 24 hours	Half of the three-quarters of the needs of the first 24 hours 20% - 60% of the calculated plasma volume	**2,000 ml**
Parkland and Baxter	Lactated Ringer's 4 ml/Kg/% of the burn					
Hypertonic sodium solution	Volume to maintain urine output at 30 ml/h (the liquid contains 250 mEq Na/liter).			One third of the oral saline solution, up to a limit of 3,500 ml.		
Brooke modified	Lactated Ringer's 2 ml/Kg/% of the burn				0.3 - 0.5ml/Kg/% of burn	**Objective: to maintain adequate urine output**
Burnett, Burn Center.	**Isotonic or hypertonic alkaline solution/% of burn/Kg**			**Keep the MS** n 51/4	**Colloid 0.5 ml/% of burn /Kg**	**D5W (% burn) (total body surface, m2)**

Source: HUDAK, Carolyn M.; GALLO, Bàrbara M. - Intensive Care Nursing - A Holistic Approach, Rio de Janeiro, RJ, Ed.:Guanabara Koogan, 1997.

6.3. ANNEX 3: Triage of Burn Victim Patients

Sorting	Outpatients	General Hospital	Burn Therapy Unit
2nd and 3rd degree burns in patients aged between 10 and 50.	Less than 10% SCQ.	Less than 20% SCQ.	**Greater than 20% SCQ.**
2nd and 3rd degree burns in patients of other age groups.	Less than 5% SCQ.	Less than 10% SCQ.	**Greater than 20% SCQ.**
3rd degree burns at any age.	"Avoid"	Less than 5% SCQ.	**Greater than 5% SCQ.**
2nd and 3rd degree burns involving the hands, face, feet and perineum.	"Never"	"Avoid"	**"Prefer"**

Electrical burns.	"Never"	"Avoid"	**"Prefer"**
Chemical burns.	"Never"	"Avoid"	**"Prefer"**
Freezing.	"Never"	"Avoid"	**"Prefer"**
Association with previous pathologies.	"Never"	"Avoid"	**"Prefer"**
Associated with fractures and polytraumas.	**"Never"**	**"Avoid"**	**"Prefer"**

Source: TABORDA, Alexandre César et.al - Curso de Atendimento Avançado em Urgência e Emergência, São Paulo, 2004 - handout.

6.4. ANNEX 4: Characteristics of the most common burns.

Burns Electrical	• Cardiac monitoring for 24 - 48 hours. • Injuries to the extremities should be monitored continuously for compartment syndrome. • Urinary monitoring for myoglobinuria and acidosis • Late ocular and neurological sequelae. • They tend to be progressive, especially in the limbs. • They have an entrance and exit door.
Burns Chemistry	• Continuous irrigation with running water and irrigation of the eyeball with isotonic solution for 30 minutes, as they cause progressive damage until the agent is completely removed. • Until proven otherwise, they should be considered deep burns. • Exposure to hydrofluoric acid can lead to severe hypocalcemia.
Liquid burns	• Exposed areas tend to be more superficial than those with clothing. • They tend to have an irregular shape and a "runny" appearance. • Immersion burns tend to be deep and severe.
Contact burns	• They are usually limited in length, but deep. • When they lose their consistency, they tend to be very deep.

Source: Knobel E. Cuidados ao paciente critico. Sao Paulo, Atheneu, 2006.

6.5. ANNEX 5: Burn depth table.

Depth	Tissues affected	Common causes	Features	Pain	Healing

Partial thickness (1st degree)	Minimal epithelial injury	Sun	Dry No vesicles Rosy red Whitens with pressure	Painful	**About five days**
Partial superficial thickness (2nd degree)	Epidermis. Dermis minima	Hot liquids light	Ùmida Reddish pink dotted Vesicle Some discoloration	Pain Hyperesthesia	**About 21 days, minimal fibrosis.**
Partial thickness Deep dermal (2nd degree)	The whole epidermis, part of the dermis, sweat glands and hairy glands lined with integral epidermis.	Hotter solids, flames and intense radiation damage.	Dry Clear No discoloration	Pressure sensitive	**Prolonged; late hypertrophic fibrosis; marked formation of contractures.**
Total thickness (3rd degree)	**All of the above and portions of subcutaneous fat; it can affect connective tissue, muscle, bone.**	**Continuous flame, electric, chemical and steam.**	**Avascular; presence of cracks; pale yellow to charred brown.**	**Little pain**	**It doesn't self-generate;** **needs grafting.**

Source: Sassine SW, Moura DF Jr, Laselva CR. Burns. In: Knobel E. Terapia Intensiva - Enfermagem. Sao Paulo, Atheneu, 2006.

6.6 . ANNEX 6 Nursing procedures in the acute phase.

Actions	Considerations
Install the patient in a private bed and promote isolation by contact precautions	The use of aprons, procedure gloves and masks is recommended
Perform a detailed physical examination on patient admission	The major burn victim may be a victim of polytrauma, so the use of the usual trauma assessment is required.
Examine the cervical region for subcutaneous emphysema, pain, vein distension, wounds and bruises.	These signs can help diagnose tension pneumothorax and cardiac tamponade

Examine the thoracic region for symmetry, expandability, wounds, abrasions, deformities and the presence of subcutaneous emphysema. Examine the abdomen and pelvis: Evaluate wounds, abrasions, flaccidity, pain on palpation and presence of hydroaerial noises	
Assess the stability of the pelvic bones, deformities suggestive of fractures, presence of urethral, vaginal or anal bleeding	
Examine upper limbs and lower limbs. Observe for wounds, fractures, motor or sensory deficits, pulse, hematoma, edema, pain, skin color, temperature and perfusion.	
Assess the occurrence of inhalation injury. The presence of scorched nasal hairs, burns around the mouth or neck, expectoration of soot can be indicative.	Data suggestive of inhalation injury associated with acute respiratory failure may determine the need for tracheal intubation.
when the event occurred	
Evaluate signals looking for instabilities to be corrected	
Apply the Glasgow Coma Scale, diameter assessment and papillary photoreaction	
Administer tetanus toxoid	According to doctor's prescription or institutional protocol
Always mobilize the major burn patient en bloc	
Maintain patent upper airways and promote mobilization or removal of pulmonary secretions	
Maintain oxygen saturation above 90%	Oxygen supply via mask or endotracheal tube
Secure the intubation cannula with a shoelace and protect the ear cartilage with a gauze pad and Micropore®.	Prevent skin damage
Permanently assess the need for sedatives and analgesia	Psychomotor agitation may be indicative of tissue

	hypoperfusion or hypoxia
Position the burnt ends upright and properly aligned	Prevents edema and sequelae of improper positioning
Encourage the patient to perform exercises with the burned extremities, whenever possible.	After prior assessment of the absence of contraindications by the surgical team
Preparing the patient for closed dressings under sedation	All procedures in the acute phase of burn injury should be performed under general anesthesia
Protect compression areas against pressure ulcers	
Perform active or passive movement every two hours, if possible	Prevents pressure ulcers
Maintain body alignment, abduction of upper limbs to 20° and lower limbs	
a 10°	
Ensure the patient is immobilized in bed, if recent grafts have been performed in the posterior region, maintaining body alignment.	Consider the need for sedation
Moisten mesh grafts with warm saline solution	Prevents adhesion
Do not apply external pressure cuff devices to burnt areas	
Cover the eye area with lubricating ointment	Prevents corneal damage and dryness
Keep patient warm with thermal blanket	Special attention during patient transportation avoiding heat
Trim hair from areas near wounds	Helps prevent infections
Perform dressings as directed by the doctor	It is recommended to maintain aseptic technique, a warm environment, adequate analgesia
Clean wounds with antimicrobial soap at least once a day	Open dressings should be carried out in stages, starting in the caudal cephalic position, ensuring that body temperature is maintained.
Assess catheter, probe and drain insertion sites twice a day	Allows early identification of infection sites

Collecting skin cultures	According to medical prescription
Pay attention to temperature equal to or greater than 38°C, and leukocytosis above 10,000/mm^3	Signs of infection
Administering enteral nutrition	The diet should be started early and the patient's tolerance to the procedure should be monitored
Weigh the patient once a day	

Source: Sassine SW, Moura DF Jr, Laselva CR. Burns. In: Knobel E. Terapia Intensiva - Enfermagem. Sao Paulo, Atheneu, 2006.

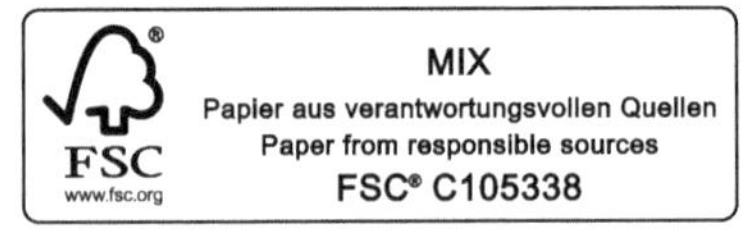

Printed by Books on Demand GmbH, Norderstedt / Germany